AOSpine Masters Series

Spinal Cord Injury and Regeneration

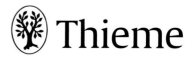

AOSpine Masters Series

Spinal Cord Injury and Regeneration

Series Editor:

Luiz Roberto Vialle, MD, PhD
Professor of Orthopedics, School of Medicine
Catholic University of Parana State
Spine Unit
Curitiba, Brazil

Guest Editors:

Michael G. Fehlings, MD, PhD, FRCSC, FACS
Head Spinal Program and Senior Scientist
McEwen Centre for Regenerative Medicine
Toronto Western Hospital
University Health Network
Professor of Neurosurgery
Vice Chair Research
Halbert Chair in Neural Repair and Regeneration
Co-Chairman Spinal Program
Division of Neurosurgery
Department of Surgery
University of Toronto
Toronto, Ontario, Canada

Norbert Weidner, MD
Professor and Chair
Spinal Cord Injury Center
Heidelberg University Hospital
Heidelberg, Germany

With 31 figures

Thieme
New York • Stuttgart • Delhi • Rio de Janeiro

Thieme Medical Publishers, Inc.
333 Seventh Ave.
New York, NY 10001

Executive Editor: William Lamsback
Managing Editor: Sarah Landis
Director, Editorial Services: Mary Jo Casey
Editorial Assistant: Haley Paskalides
Production Editor: Barbara A. Chernow
International Production Director: Andreas Schabert
Vice President, Editorial and E-Product Development: Vera Spillner
International Marketing Director: Fiona Henderson
International Sales Director: Louisa Turrell
Director of Sales, North America: Mike Roseman
Senior Vice President and Chief Operating Officer: Sarah Vanderbilt
President: Brian D. Scanlan
Compositor: Carol Pierson, Chernow Editorial Services, Inc.

Library of Congress Cataloging-in-Publication Data
Names: Vialle, Luiz Roberto, editor. | Fehlings, Michael, editor. | Weidner, Norbert, editor. | AOSpine
    International (Firm), sponsoring body.
Title: AOSspine masters series. V. 7, Spinal cord injury and regeneration / editors, Luiz Roberto Vialle,
    Michael G. Fehlings, Norbert Weidner.
Other titles: Spinal cord injury and regeneration
Description: New York : Thieme, [2016] | Includes bibliographical references and index.
Identifiers: LCCN 2016021476 (print) | LCCN 2016021669 (ebook) | ISBN 9781626232273 (alk. paper) | ISBN
    9781626232280
Subjects: | MESH: Spinal Cord Injuries—therapy | Spinal Cord Regeneration
Classification: LCC RA645.S66 (print) | LCC RA645.S66 (ebook) | NLM WL 403 | DDC 617.4/82044—dc23
LC record available at https://lccn.loc.gov/2016021476

Printed in China by Everbest Printing Ltd.
5 4 3 2 1
ISBN 978-1-62623-227-3

Also available as an e-book:
eISBN 978-1-62623-228-0

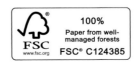

100%
Paper from well-managed forests
FSC® C124385

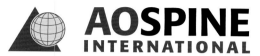

AOSpine Masters Series

Luiz Roberto Vialle, MD, PhD
Series Editor

Volume 1   Metastatic Spinal Tumors

Volume 2   Primary Spinal Tumors

Volume 3   Cervical Degenerative Conditions

Volume 4   Adult Spinal Deformities

Volume 5   Cervical Spine Trauma

Volume 6   Thoracolumbar Spine Trauma

Volume 7   Spinal Cord Injury and Regeneration

Volume 8   Back Pain

Volume 9   Pediatric Spinal Deformities

Volume 10   Spinal Infection

Contents

Series Preface ix
    Luiz Roberto Vialle

Guest Editors' Preface xi
    Michael G. Fehlings and Norbert Weidner

1 Pathobiology of Spinal Cord Injury 1
    Hiroaki Nakashima, Narihito Nagoshi, and Michael G. Fehlings

2 Assessment of Functional Status and Outcomes of Individuals with
    Traumatic Spinal Cord Injury 11
    Christian Schuld and Norbert Weidner

3 Serum and CSF Biomarkers to Predict Functional Recovery After Spinal Cord Injury 25
    Seth S. Tigchelaar and Brian K. Kwon

4 Magnetic Resonance Imaging of the Injured Spinal Cord:
    The Present and the Future 39
    Allan R. Martin, Julien Cohen-Adad, and Michael G. Fehlings

5 Acute Nonoperative Management of Traumatic Spinal Cord Injury:
    State of the Art 57
    Joshua S. Catapano, Gregory W.J. Hawryluk, and Michael G. Fehlings

6 Role and Timing of Surgery for Traumatic Spinal Cord Injury:
    What Do We Know and What Should We Do? 71
    Christopher D. Witiw and Michael G. Fehlings

7 Methylprednisolone As a Valid Option for Acute Spinal Cord Injury:
    A Reassessment of the Literature 80
    Michael G. Fehlings and Newton Cho

8 Neuroprotection of the Injured Spinal Cord: What Does the Future Hold? 89
    Christopher S. Ahuja and Michael G. Fehlings

9 Hydrogel Biomaterials in Spinal Cord Repair and Regeneration 107
    Manuel Ingo Günther, Thomas Schackel, Norbert Weidner, and Armin Blesch

10 Neural Stem Cell Transplantation for Spinal Cord Repair 122
Ina K. Simeonova, Beatrice Sandner, and Norbert Weidner

11 Strategies to Overcome the Inhibitory Environment of the Spinal Cord 132
Elizabeth J. Bradbury and Emily R. Burnside

12 Functional Electrical Stimulation and Neuromodulation Approaches to
Enhance Recovery After Spinal Cord Injury 148
César Márquez-Chin, Emilie Sagripanti, and Milos R. Popovic

13 Advanced Rehabilitation Strategies for Individuals with Traumatic Spinal
Cord Injury 163
William Z. Rymer, Sheila Burt, and Arun Jayaraman

14 Brain–Computer Interfaces to Enhance Function After Spinal Cord Injury 179
Rüdiger Rupp

Index 193

Series Preface

Spine care is advancing at a rapid pace. The challenge for today's spine care professional is to quickly synthesize the best available evidence and expert opinion in the management of spine pathologies. The AOSpine Masters Series provides just that—each volume in the series delivers pathology-focused expert opinion on procedures, diagnosis, clinical wisdom, and pitfalls, and highlights today's top research papers.

To bring the value of its masters level educational courses and academic congresses to a wider audience, AOSpine has assembled internationally recognized spine pathology leaders to develop volumes in this Masters Series as a vehicle for sharing their experiences and expertise and providing links to the literature. Each volume focuses on a current compelling and sometimes controversial topic in spine care.

The unique and efficient format of the Masters Series volumes quickly focuses the attention of the reader on the core information critical to understanding the topic, while encouraging the reader to look further into the recommended literature.

Through this approach, AOSpine is advancing spine care worldwide.

Luiz Roberto Vialle, MD, PhD

Emilie Sagripanti
Medical Student
Rehabilitation Engineering Laboratory
Toronto Rehabilitation Institute
University Health Network
Toronto, Ontario, Canada

Beatrice Sandner, MD
Postdoctoral Fellow
Spinal Cord Injury Center
Heidelberg University Hospital
Heidelberg, Germany

Thomas Schackel, MSc
Graduate Student
Spinal Cord Injury Center
Heidelberg University Hospital
Heidelberg, Germany

Christian Schuld, Dipl.-Inform. Med.
Research Associate
Spinal Cord Injury Center
Heidelberg University Hospital
Heidelberg, Germany

Ina K. Simeonova, MSc
PhD Candidate
Spinal Cord Injury Center
Heidelberg University Hospital
Heidelberg, Germany

Seth S. Tigchelaar, BSc
PhD Candidate
Department of Neuroscience
University of British Columbia
Vancouver, British Columbia, Canada

Norbert Weidner, MD
Professor and Chair
Spinal Cord Injury Center
Heidelberg University Hospital
Heidelberg, Germany

Christopher D. Witiw, MD
Neurosurgery Resident
Department of Surgery
Division of Neurosurgery
University of Toronto
Toronto, Ontario, Canada

1

Pathobiology of Spinal Cord Injury

Hiroaki Nakashima, Narihito Nagoshi, and Michael G. Fehlings

◼ Introduction

Spinal cord injury (SCI) is a devastating event often resulting in neurologic deficit with social, economic and emotional repercussions for patients. It is estimated that acute traumatic SCI has an annual incidence of 15 to 40 cases per million. SCI costs society in excess of $7 billion annually,[1] and contributes significantly to human suffering related to impaired ambulation and sexual and sphincter dysfunction.

The pathobiology of spinal cord damage following SCI is conceptually constituted of primary and secondary injury phases (**Table 1.1**).[1,2] The initial mechanical disruption to the spinal cord constitutes the primary phase. The secondary injury refers to a wide range of downstream progressive events including vascular dysfunction, edema, ischemia, excitotoxicity, and free radical production. This secondary injury phase continues after the primary injury has ceased and can last for weeks or even years. The cellular and molecular processes related to secondary injury are complex and alter over time, which is of great relevance to the timing of therapeutics that might be administered. This chapter summarizes our knowledge of SCI pathobiology using knowledge gleaned from our rodent model.

◼ Primary Spinal Cord Injury

Primary SCI occurs at the time of injury as a result of the physical forces impacting on the spinal cord and is the key determinant of the severity of spinal cord damage. SCI is most commonly the result of displaced elements of the vertebral column, including intervertebral disks and ligaments, which then exert force on the cord, causing both immediate SCI and often sustained compression.[1] Sustained compression of the spinal cord is observed in many cases after the initial impact of the injury. The most common primary injury mechanisms are shear, stretch, and, in particular, contusive and compressive forces.[1,2] In addition, spinal cord laceration has been observed in a small number of cases due to vertebral bone fragments or from violence involving weapons. These forces disrupt axons, blood vessels, and cell membranes. Complete transection of the spinal cord is a rare occurrence even in cases with complete paralysis. In cases with complete paralysis, viable axons are usually found around the lesion site, often occupying a subpial rim. However, the reason for dysfunction is the extensive loss of oligodendrocytes and their myelin sheaths.[3] The existence of these spared axons crossing the injury site is seen as a potential therapeutic

Table 1.1 Timeline of Spinal Cord Injury Phases

Injury Phase		Key Processes and Events
Primary	Immediate (< 2 hours)	Traumatic physical injury Axon severing Gray matter hemorrhage and ischemia Microglial activation Necrotic cell death Release of proinflammatory factors: IL-1β, TNF-α, IL-6, and others
Secondary	Early acute (< 48 hours)	Continued hemorrhage, ischemia, and necrosis Neutrophil invasion Free radical production: lipid peroxidation Increased BSCB permeability Glutamate-mediated excitotoxicity Neutrophil invasion Vasogenic and cytoxic edema Oligodendrocyte death and early demyelination Neuronal death
	Subacute (< 14 days)	Maximal phagocytic response Macrophage infiltration Initiation of reactive gliosis and glial scar formation BSCB repair and resolution of edema
	Intermediate (< 6 months)	Continued glial scar formation Cyst formation Lesion stabilization
	Chronic (> 6 months)	Prolonged wallerian degeneration Potential structural and functional plasticity of spared spinal cord tissue

target for the improvement of neurologic function, and represents the neural substrate on which many emerging therapeutic strategies will act.

In recent decades, central cord injury has become more prevalent, and can occur in patients of all ages. It entails motor impairment of the upper extremities that is more pronounced than that of the lower extremities. This injury occurs via different mechanisms in younger versus older patients. Younger patients are typically affected as a result of severe spinal column injury.[4] In contrast, older patients with long-standing cervical spondylosis do not typically suffer bony injuries. Instead hyperextension injury results in trauma to the cord. In this pathology, primary injury results from sudden "pinching" of spinal cord between a posterior buckled ligamentum flavum and anterior osteophytes and disk regions. Central cord injury is more common in older patients, where the incidence of cervical spondylosis or acquired spinal stenosis due to degenerative changes is higher.

It is often said that clinicians cannot affect the occurrence of primary SCI, but education, safety legislation, and technology can have a significant impact on the incidence and severity of this primary injury. As a result of these developments, both the incidence and severity of SCI tends to be decreasing. For example, prehospital use of a cervical collar in trauma patients can potentially reduce primary damage to the spinal cord, and airbag technology in motor vehicles has reduced lumbosacral injuries in recent years.

■ Secondary Spinal Cord Injury

The initial trauma to the spinal cord triggers a series of systemic, cellular, and molecular cas-

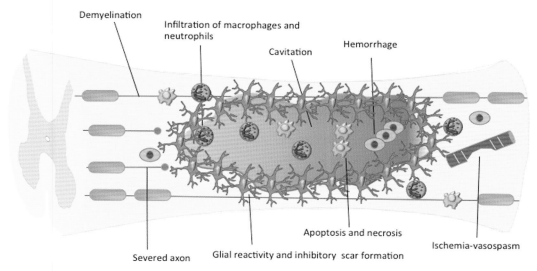

Demyelination

Infiltration of macrophages and
neutrophils

Cavitation

Hemorrhage

Apoptosis and necrosis

Ischemia-vasospasm

Severed axon   Glial reactivity and inhibitory scar formation

Fig. 1.1 Pathophysiological events occurring after spinal cord injury (SCI), including the acute, subacute, and chronic phases.

cades that expand the lesion from the primary injury site into adjacent white matter and gray matter. This delayed, progressive, and protracted tissue injury is known as secondary spinal cord injury (**Fig. 1.1**). In general, the force of the primary injury determines the size and extent of the ensuing hemorrhage, which in turn dictates the extent of ischemia and other aspects of secondary damage. These secondary SCI processes, in addition to ischemia, include free radicals and oxidative stress, ionic dysregulation and glutamate excitotoxity, mitochondrial dysfunction, blood–spinal cord barrier (BSCB) compromise, neuroinflammation, and cell death and apoptosis.[5]

Changes in Spinal Cord Blood Flow and Ischemia

The traumatized spinal cord in the acute stage shows severe hemorrhages predominantly in the gray matter, leading to hemorrhagic necrosis and central myelomalacia at the lesion site, according to a study by Tator and Fehlings.[6] But they found no evidence of complete occlusion of any large spinal arteries, whereas occluded intramedullary veins were identified in the white column. Also, measurement of spinal

cord blood flow after acute injury demonstrated that there is a major reduction of blood flow in the parenchyma of the injured spinal cord. Disruption of the microvasculature, loss of normal autoregulatory mechanisms, the occurrence of vasospasm and thrombosis, and accumulation of fluid and edema contribute to this ischemia. This ischemic status enhances the cascade of secondary injury processes, such as free radical formation, glutamate-mediated excitotoxicity, ionic dysregulation, inflammatory response, and disruption of the BSCB. These processes are all interrelated, and eventually lead to axonal degeneration and cell death.

Free Radicals and Oxidative Stress

Free radicals are highly reactive molecules possessing an unpaired electron on their outer shell. This unpaired electron provides high chemical reactivity. The term *reactive oxygen species* (ROS) includes some kinds of free radicals, such as superoxide and hydrogen peroxide. Free radicals and ROS are generated during the process of oxidative metabolism in mitochondria, and under normal biological conditions, their activity is suppressed by endogenous antioxidants.

However, this oxidant/antioxidant balance is disrupted during the secondary injury process, leading to oxidative stress. The excessive formation of free radicals and ROS results from mitochondrial dysfunction, increasing intracellular calcium levels, arachidonic acid breakdown, and activation of inducible nitric oxide synthase.[7] Neutrophil infiltration into the lesion site also contributes as a source of ROS through oxidative bursts. Free radicals and ROS attack biological molecules such as proteins, DNA, and lipids by oxidation. These processes enhance adverse mechanisms of neural injury, such as spinal cord hypoperfusion, the development of edema, axonal conduction failure, and breakdown of energy metabolism with accompanying necrotic and apoptotic cell death.[8]

Ionic Dysregulation and Glutamate Excitotoxicity

Ionic dysregulation and glutamate excitotoxicity play key roles in the evolution of the secondary injury following acute SCI.[5] After SCI, neuronal ionic balance is disrupted, and intracellular sodium concentration increases as a result of trauma-induced activation of voltage-gated sodium channels. These increases in sodium concentration in neuronal cells promote cellular swelling and the development of intracellular acidosis and cytotoxic edema through increased entry of protons via sodium–proton exchangers. In addition, concomitant influx of calcium ions also occurs with the increase of sodium concentration via the sodium–calcium exchanger, inducing extracellular release of the excitatory neurotransmitter glutamate in presynaptic neurons. Impaired glutamate reuptake by astrocytes through dysfunction in glutamate transporters also contributes to increased extracellular glutamates. High concentrations of glutamic acid can accumulate in the synaptic cleft and promote excitotoxicity. The presence of excitotoxic concentrations of glutamic acid in the cleft results in excessive stimulation of excitatory amino acid receptors on the postsynaptic cell, leading to the entry of sodium and calcium ions through N-methyl-D-aspartic acid (NMDA) and non-NMDA receptors. The excessive influx of ions depolarizes the postsynaptic cells and triggers the activation of voltage-gated sodium and calcium channels, amplifying the depolarization. This process eventually leads to edema and apoptotic death in the postsynaptic neural axons.

One of the therapeutic strategies for attenuating ionic imbalance is to block the sodium channels and prevent the excessive influx of various ions with the use of pharmacological drugs. Riluzole, a sodium channel blocker, is a promising agent to diminish neurologic tissue destruction and attenuate the secondary injury, and has been demonstrated to be effective in laboratory research in rodent models.[9] Currently, an international, multicenter phase II/III clinical trial, the Riluzole in Acute Spinal Cord Injury Study (RISCIS; NCT01597518), is ongoing in patients with acute SCI.[10]

Mitochondrial Dysfunction

In general, mitochondria play an important role in oxidative phosphorylation and adenosine triphosphate (ATP) supply. ATP production is controlled by mitochondrial calcium ions. Mitochondria act as high-capacity calcium sinks, taking up excessive calcium ions to maintain homeostatic levels of calcium concentration within the cytosol.[11] After SCI, however, the aforementioned excessive influx of calcium ions into postsynaptic cells results in the formation of mitochondrial permeability transition pores (mPTPs). Once an mPTP opens, molecules and concomitant water can enter the mitochondria, and this influx causes the mitochondria to swell as they achieve equilibrium with the cytosol. This matrix swelling eventually leads to rupture of the mitochondrial membrane. Disruption of the membrane releases ROS, accumulated calcium ions, and proapoptotic molecules (e.g., cytochrome c, SMAC/DIABLO, and apoptosis-inducing factor). These substances lead to activation of cell death pathways, such as apoptosis, autophagy, and necrosis.

Blood–Spinal Cord Barrier Compromise

The BSCB anatomically consists of endothelial cells linked with tight junctions and their accessory structures, including astrocytic end-feet processes, pericytes, and the basement membrane. This barrier has an important function in protecting the spinal cord parenchyma from exogenous infection and toxins, and in regulating the transport of molecules in and out of the spinal cord. The BSCB provides an optimal environment for neuronal activities by regulating nutrients and neurotoxins.

The primary injury in SCI causes vascular disruption and breakdown of the BSCB. Further BSCB compromise results from the degeneration of endothelial tight junction proteins, and the disappearance of astrocytic end feet due to cell death. Progression of BSCB permeability enables cellular and molecular inflammatory mediators to intrude into the parenchyma of the spinal cord, initiating and expanding the secondary injury. The time taken until the BSCB is reestablished has variously been reported as between 14 and 56 days postinjury.[12] The prolonged permeability of the BSCB results from upregulation of inflammatory cytokines such as interleukin-1β (IL-1β) and tumor necrosis factor-α (TNF-α), and other signaling molecules such as ROS, histamines, and nitric oxide. The permeability also contributes to the development of edema. Some angiogenetic factors, such as vascular endothelial growth factor and hepatocyte growth factor, contribute to neovascularization and BSCB repair.

Neuroinflammation

The inflammatory response initiated after SCI is a complex series of cellular and molecular events with systematic and local mediators.[13] The process involves orchestrated activation of various factors including phagocytic cells (microglia, macrophages, neutrophils), lymphocytes, and soluble mediators (chemokines, cytokines, complement). The inflammatory processes vary depending on animal species and strains. The SCI model used and the level of injury also contribute to differences in the inflammatory response. Inflammation has both beneficial and detrimental roles in removing cellular debris, which aids tissue repair, and in propagating the secondary damage processes.

Within hours after SCI, resident microglia are activated, due to vascular disruption and loss of homeostasis, and migrate toward the lesion site. Microglia react to the injury by changing their morphology and releasing cytokines such as IL-1, IL-6, TNF-α, free radicals and nitric oxide, and chemokines such as leukotrienes and prostaglandins.[13] These mediators play roles in recruiting inflammatory cells and modulating protein expression in neuronal and glial cells, and lead to neurotoxicity and myelin damage. Microglia may also contribute to debris phagocytosis rather than apoptosis induction.

Increasing the permeability of the BSCB after the primary injury, neutrophils infiltrate into the injured spinal cord. They accumulate in the lesion site starting hours after injury and continuing up to 3 days after SCI, and are rapidly cleared in the first week. Neutrophils release matrix metalloproteinases (MMPs) and myeloperoxidase, which lead to ROS production and lipid peroxidation.

Monocyte-derived macrophages are recruited to the lesion site from peripheral circulation a few days after SCI. Unlike neutrophils, macrophages stay in the injured spinal cord for months in rodents and years in humans.[14] The macrophages are indistinguishable from resident microglia when examined histologically, and show similar cytokine expression profiles. Macrophages are believed to have both beneficial and detrimental roles. Long-lasting release of proinflammatory cytokines, free radicals, and proteases by macrophages may contribute to neuronal and glial toxicity. Depletion of macrophages, or inhibition of their function, contributes to neural repair and recovery of neurologic function.[14] Conversely, activation of macrophages may also protect and repair the injured spinal cord to modulate glutamate excitotoxicity and to produce growth factors essential for neuronal survival and tissue repair.[14]

Lymphocytes infiltrate the spinal cord maximally between 3 and 7 days after injury in response to the cytokine/chemokine signals from activated microglia/macrophages. T-lymphocytes recognize myelin basic protein (MBP), and amplify the reactions. These autoimmune responses aggravate demyelination and axonal degeneration, and increase the size of the lesion site. Again, however, lymphocytes may also play an important role in repairing the injured spinal cord. Lymphocytes can secrete neurotrophins such as brain-derived neurotrophic factor (BDNF) and insulin-like growth factor-1 (IGF-1), and active immunization with MBP promotes functional recovery.[15]

Necrotic and Apoptotic Cell Death

Following SCI, cell death can occur due to necrosis or apoptosis. The pathway of cell death is dictated by the intensity of the cellular insult. Necrosis occurs as a result of physical damage or disease. In this "accidental" form of cell death, intracellular contents are released into the extracellular matrix, causing an inflammatory reaction. In contrast, apoptotic cell death is a form of programmed cell death that involves cell shrinkage, genomic fragmentation, and karyorrhexis.[13] Acute cell death after SCI is necrosis in most cases, whereas delayed cell death is caused by apoptosis. Necrosis can cause physical and chemical membrane damage and excessive accumulation of intracellular ROS. Apoptosis is induced by mitochondrial dysfunction with cytochrome c release and caspase-9 activation. The other signaling pathways of apoptosis include activation of death receptors such as TNFR, Fas, p75, and DR3.[13] Expression of Fas and p75 receptors is seen in oligodendrocytes, astrocytes, and microglia; downstream, caspase-3 and -8 lead to apoptosis.[16]

Demyelination

Oligodendrocytes are myelinating cells in the central nervous system (CNS), and they play a critical role in promoting transduction of action potentials along neuronal axons. In addition, oligodendrocytes protect neurons with trophic, metabolic, and structural support. After SCI, the communication between myelinating oligodendrocytes and neuronal axons is disrupted. During the acute and subacute stages of secondary damage, inflammation, ischemia, free radical formation, excitotoxicity, and dysregulation of ion equilibrium contribute to the death of oligodendrocytes, leading to myelin loss and dysfunction.[17] Apoptosis predominantly occurs in nonneuronal cells such as oligodendrocytes between 24 hours and 7 days following injury, and this event leads eventually to anterograde neurodegeneration. As a result, saltatory conduction is lost, and axonal degeneration occurs over time. Spontaneous remyelination occurs after injury, but is insufficient for repair. Endogenous oligodendrocyte precursor cells (OPCs) proliferate in response to the SCI, and migrate toward the lesion site. The migrated OPCs differentiate into astrocytes to contribute to glial scar formation. Although some OPCs can also produce oligodendrocytes, their maturation is not complete. Recent findings suggest that myelinating Schwann cells at the lesion site are derived not only from peripheral nerve roots but also from the residual OPCs.[18] Overall, the activation of endogenous OPCs and enhancement of their myelination potential using external factors may be an optimal strategy for functional recovery after SCI. Another strategy with exciting potential is cell transplantation therapy, in which OPCs are cultured and harvested from various cellular sources, such as induced pluripotent stem cells (iPSCs), embryonic stem cells, or somatic neural stem cells. The efficacy of OPC transplantation has already been demonstrated in laboratory research.

▪ Limited Regenerative Capacity of the Central Nervous System

In the first description of injured neurons, by Santiago Ramón y Cajal in 1928, it was thought that the injured neurons themselves in the CNS had limited axonal regenerative capacity due to the dystrophic "end-balls" he observed at the end of the axon, which he believed were no longer capable of regeneration.[19] However, later reports indicated the possibility that these dystrophic end-balls were not a sign of axonal regeneration failure, but rather an active structure occurring postinjury.[19] In fact, axonal regeneration is observed in the CNS for months after an injury. Unfortunately, these regenerative responses are less than those seen in peripheral axons. Axonal regeneration depends on several regenerative molecules including GAP-43, neurotrophins, cyclic adenosine monophosphate (cAMP) and tubulins. The expression levels of these genes are lower in the CNS following injury than in the peripheral nervous system (PNS), and this results in the lower regeneration capacity of the CNS.[20]

Furthermore, recent scientific advances have suggested that many inhibitory repulsive guidance molecules related to axonal pathfinding during development continue to be found in adults and could reduce axon regeneration after injury. In addition, the glial environment of the adult CNS, which is different from that of the PNS or embryonic nervous system, affects axonal regeneration. The nerve fibers in the CNS are ensheathed by oligodendrocytes, but they are exposed to myelin-associated inhibitors after injury. In addition, a glial scar consisting of reactive astrocytes could act as an additional barrier and thus inhibit axon regrowth.

Myelin-Associated Inhibitory Molecules[19]

The specific environment related to myelin in the CNS is one of the biggest factors contributing to the inhibition of regeneration after injury, and it is suspected that there is a specific inhibitor of axonal growth inherent in myelin. In fact, cultured sympathetic ganglion neurons extend their neurites on myelin in the PNS but not in the CNS. Nogo is one of the first reported inhibitors inherent to myelin, which triggers growth cone collapse. Other studies led to the identification of several other myelin-associated components that can inhibit axon outgrowth in vitro, including myelin-associated

glycoprotein (MAG), oligodendrocyte myelin glycoprotein (OMgp), semaphorin 4D, and ephrin B3.

Although Nogo, MAG, and OMgp lack sequence homologies, they all bind to the Nogo receptor (NgR) (**Fig. 1.2**). This NgR is glycosylphosphatidyl-inositol (GPI) linked, lacks an intracellular domain, and transduces intracellular inhibitory signals by forming co-receptor complexes with the TNF receptor family proteins such as p75 and TROY, as well as LINGO-1. These complexes activate the Rho/Rock pathway, leading to decreased growth cone mobility and growth cone collapse.

Glial Scarring and Chondroitin Sulfate Proteoglycans[19]

The glial scar is another major element contributing to the inhibition of regeneration within the CNS. This glial scarring is a result of the recruitment of microglia, oligodendrocyte precursors, meningeal cells, and astrocytes to the lesion site. Some of these responses have beneficial qualities. Reactive astrocytes reestablish ionic homeostasis and the integrity of the BSCB, which is important for the resolution of edema and in limiting the infiltration of immune cells. Although much of the glial scar contains inhibitory chondroitin sulfate proteoglycans, there are regions that are rich in growth promoting extracellular matrix (ECM) molecules such as laminin and fibronectin. Astrocytes are also thought to supply neurons with energy and to help in the release of growth factors and beneficial cytokines.

In contrast, astrocytes at the lesion core often begin to display a hypertrophic reactive phenotype, forming a chemical barrier by secreting several growth inhibitory chondroitin sulfate proteoglycans (CSPGs), which include neurocan, versican, aggrecan, brevican, phosphacan, and NG2. These form a family of molecules characterized by a protein core to which large, highly sulfated glycosaminoglycan (GAG) chains are attached. It is associated with fibroblast infiltration and the deposition of inhibitory ECM molecules. These molecules function as chemical barriers to axonal regeneration in the same fashion as myelin inhibitors.

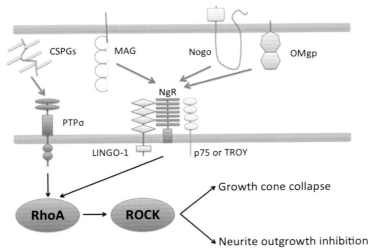

Fig. 1.2 Molecular mechanisms of myelin inhibition and potential for therapeutic intervention. The Nogo 66 peptide of Nogo A binds to the Nogo receptor (NgR) along with myelin-associated glycoprotein (MAG) and oligodendrocyte myelin glycoprotein (OMgp). NgR lacks a cytoplasmic domain and must interact with the tumor necrosis factor (TNF) receptor family proteins to transduce signals intracellularly. Ligand-receptor binding activates RhoA, and RhoA then activates Rho kinase (ROCK). ROCK has growth inhibitory effects on the actin cytoskeleton, showing growth cone collapse and neurite outgrowth inhibition. CSPGs, chondroitin sulfate proteoglycans; PTP, permeability transition pore.

This inhibitory activity of CSPGs depends on the GAG components. Chondroitinase ABC (ChABC) is known as an enzyme that removes GAG chains from the protein core and eliminates this inhibition. Thus, ChABC is expected to contribute to the reduction of glial scarring. Recently, the receptor for CSPGs, PTPsigma was discovered; this is a transmembrane tyrosine phosphatase. CSPGs also signal through the Rho/Rock pathway just as in Nogo, MAG, and OMgp. This downstream signaling cascade could be a therapeutic target to reduce glial scarring and thus remove a barrier to axonal regeneration.

Limited Progenitor Cell Proliferation[21]

Endogenous stem/progenitor cells have been identified in the adult mammalian spinal cord. In intact spinal cords, latent neural stem cells are found in the ependymal layer around the central canal and an intact corticospinal tract. In the intact spinal cord, progenitor cells rarely divide; however, these ependymal cells start dividing rapidly after SCI. Half of them become astrocytes in the glial scar, and a small number of them become oligodendrocytes myelinating axons. Unfortunately, this native adult neurogenesis is insufficient for robust neural repair.

▦ Chapter Summary

Spinal cord injury is a debilitating condition that is biphasic in nature with a complex series of secondary responses occurring after the initial primary injury. The most common types of primary injuries in humans are contusion or impact/compression of the spinal cord following a fracture-dislocation of the vertebral column or a burst fracture. Damage from the primary mechanical trauma causes local edema, ischemia, hemorrhage, necrosis, laceration of tissue, and release of proinflammatory factors. The secondary phases of the various pathophysiological processes exacerbate the initial damage, whereas endogenous efforts to facilitate healing and regeneration struggle to succeed. These secondary SCI processes include ischemia, free radicals and oxidative stress, ionic dysregulation and glutamate excitotoxicity, mitochondrial dysfunction, blood–spinal cord barrier compromise, neuroinflammation, and cell death and apoptosis.

Substantial tissue loss occurs after major SCI, and this results in a fluid-filled cavity in the center of the cord at the site of injury that may even enlarge over time, resulting in further tissue damage. In addition, myelin-related inhibitory molecules, such as Nogo, MAG, or OMgp, activate the Rho pathway in the injured cord. The glial scar, made up of chondroitin sulfate proteoglycans, is formed by reactive astrocytes, resulting in a physical and chemical barrier to regeneration. Spatial and temporal dynamics of these secondary mediators are central to SCI pathobiology, which was a recurring theme in this chapter. Although there have been advances in the medical and surgical management for SCI, there continues to be a significant need for effective neuroprotective and neuroregenerative therapeutic strategies. A deep understanding of the SCI pathophysiology contributing to the progression of an individual's unique injury will help the development of successful treatment paradigms.

Pearls

- Spinal cord injury is a debilitating condition resulting in a biphasic injury process, which is divided into the primary and secondary injury phases.
- Primary damage resulting from trauma causes local edema, ischemia, hemorrhage, necrosis, and laceration of tissue.
- The secondary phases that follow exacerbate the initial damage for several months.
- These secondary SCI processes include ischemia, free radicals and oxidative stress, ionic dysregulation and glutamate excitotoxicity, mitochondrial dysfunction, blood–spinal cord barrier compromise, neuroinflammation, and cell death and apoptosis.
- Myelin-related inhibitory molecules are upregulated, and a glial scar is formed by reactive astrocytes around the injury site, resulting in a physical and chemical barrier to regeneration.

Pitfalls

- Primary injury can be reduced by prehospital use of a cervical collar and by advances in airbag technology.
- We have yet to elucidate all the mechanisms involved in the secondary injury.
- We need to know more about neuroinflammation and the Rho pathway to develop therapeutics to improve patient outcomes.
- Cell transplantation therapy could overcome the limited endogenous progenitor cell proliferation after spinal cord injury.

References
Five Must-Read References

1. Sekhon LH, Fehlings MG. Epidemiology, demographics, and pathophysiology of acute spinal cord injury. Spine 2001;26(24, Suppl):S2–S12
2. Rowland JW, Hawryluk GW, Kwon B, Fehlings MG. Current status of acute spinal cord injury pathophysiology and emerging therapies: promise on the horizon. Neurosurg Focus 2008;25:E2
3. Totoiu MO, Keirstead HS. Spinal cord injury is accompanied by chronic progressive demyelination. J Comp Neurol 2005;486:373–383
4. van Middendorp JJ, Pouw MH, Hayes KC, et al; EM-SCI Study Group Collaborators. Diagnostic criteria of traumatic central cord syndrome. Part 2: a questionnaire survey among spine specialists. Spinal Cord 2010; 48:657–663
5. Schwartz G, Fehlings MG. Secondary injury mechanisms of spinal cord trauma: a novel therapeutic approach for the management of secondary pathophysiology with the sodium channel blocker riluzole. Prog Brain Res 2002;137:177–190
6. Tator CH, Fehlings MG. Review of the secondary injury theory of acute spinal cord trauma with emphasis on vascular mechanisms. J Neurosurg 1991;75:15–26
7. McTigue DM. Potential therapeutic targets for PPAR-gamma after spinal cord injury. PPAR Res 2008; 2008:517162
8. Bao F, Liu D. Peroxynitrite generated in the rat spinal cord induces apoptotic cell death and activates caspase-3. Neuroscience 2003;116:59–70

9. Wu Y, Satkunendrarajah K, Teng Y, Chow DS, Buttigieg J, Fehlings MG. Delayed post-injury administration of riluzole is neuroprotective in a preclinical rodent model of cervical spinal cord injury. J Neurotrauma 2013;30:441–452

10. Fehlings MG, Nakashima H, Nagoshi N, Chow DS, Grossman RG, Kopjar B. Rationale, design and critical end points for the Riluzole in Acute Spinal Cord Injury Study (RISCIS): a randomized, double-blinded, placebo-controlled parallel multi-center trial. Spinal Cord 2016;54:8–15

11. McEwen ML, Sullivan PG, Rabchevsky AG, Springer JE. Targeting mitochondrial function for the treatment of acute spinal cord injury. Neurotherapeutics 2011; 8:168–179

12. Bartanusz V, Jezova D, Alajajian B, Digicaylioglu M. The blood-spinal cord barrier: morphology and clinical implications. Ann Neurol 2011;70:194–206

13. Hausmann ON. Post-traumatic inflammation following spinal cord injury. Spinal Cord 2003;41:369–378

14. Donnelly DJ, Popovich PG. Inflammation and its role in neuroprotection, axonal regeneration and functional recovery after spinal cord injury. Exp Neurol 2008;209:378–388

15. Hauben E, Butovsky O, Nevo U, et al. Passive or active immunization with myelin basic protein promotes recovery from spinal cord contusion. J Neurosci 2000;20:6421–6430

16. Casha S, Yu WR, Fehlings MG. Oligodendroglial apoptosis occurs along degenerating axons and is associated with FAS and p75 expression following spinal cord injury in the rat. Neuroscience 2001;103:203–218

17. Papastefanaki F, Matsas R. From demyelination to remyelination: the road toward therapies for spinal cord injury. Glia 2015;63:1101–1125

18. Zawadzka M, Rivers LE, Fancy SP, et al. CNS-resident glial progenitor/stem cells produce Schwann cells as well as oligodendrocytes during repair of CNS demyelination. Cell Stem Cell 2010;6:578–590

19. Yiu G, He Z. Glial inhibition of CNS axon regeneration. Nat Rev Neurosci 2006;7:617–627

20. Hunt D, Hossain-Ibrahim K, Mason MR, et al. ATF3 upregulation in glia during wallerian degeneration: differential expression in peripheral nerves and CNS white matter. BMC Neurosci 2004;5:9

21. Stenudd M, Sabelström H, Frisén J. Role of endogenous neural stem cells in spinal cord injury and repair. JAMA Neurol 2015;72:235–237

2

Assessment of Functional Status and Outcomes of Individuals with Traumatic Spinal Cord Injury

Christian Schuld and Norbert Weidner

▤ Introduction

High-quality outcome measures play an important role in clinical research,[1] for which they serve as inclusion/exclusion criteria as well as stratification, subgrouping, and primary and secondary outcome measures. Outcome measures also enable health care professionals to describe, predict, and evaluate findings, so as to provide benchmarks, summarize change, and contribute to the identification of meaningful treatment goals for individuals with spinal cord injury (SCI). Therefore, outcome measures can play an important role in providing quantifiable information in clinical communication. Accordingly, they also support clinicians in their daily routine by (1) providing prognostic information by means of an early assessment after injury; (2) enabling the tailoring of individualized rehabilitation plans (e.g., compensatory versus restorative approaches, length of stay prediction, and adaptive equipment need); (3) facilitating short-term therapy planning (force training versus coordination, etc.); and (4) enabling the ability to evaluate the success of rehabilitation interventions.

▤ Quality of Outcome Measures

Key concepts in classical testing theory and psychometrics science are reliability and validity. *Reliability,* or more precisely test-retest reliability, measures the degree of consistency or agreement of repeated assessments of the same individual.[2] A distinction is made between intrarater reliability and interrater reliability. For the determination of intrarater reliability, the assessment is repeated by the same rater, whereas for interrater reliability, multiple raters assess the same individual. Reliability can be expressed by intraclass correlation coefficients (ICC) or kappa statistics for nominal or categorical scores. A common interpretation of the kappa agreement coefficient κ is as follows: poor (< 0), slight (0–0.2), fair (0.21–0.4), moderate (0.41–0.6), substantial (0.61–0.8), and almost perfect (> 0.8).[3]

Reliability is the prerequisite of validity. More specifically, reliability is necessary, but not sufficient, for validity. *Validity* is defined as the extent to which an assessment measures what it intends or purports to measure.[4] Validity comes in different variants.

Content validity verifies that the method of measurement actually measures what it is expected to measure. This verification includes evaluation of the measurement aims, the target population, clear concepts (e.g., capacity versus performance in physical functioning), item selection (the target population should be involved in item selection), as well as item reduction.[5] Item reduction keeps the assessment short by removing statistically unnecessary items.

Criterion validity refers to the extent to which scores on a particular instrument relate to a gold standard.[5] Without a gold standard, the criterion validity cannot be evaluated. Unfortunately, this is often the case in the field of spinal cord medicine. In this situation, less powerful methods are used to provide evidence of validity.

Construct validity refers to how well a test measures the constructs that it was designed to measure.[4] For new clinical outcome measures, which are in the process of validation, the new assessment and the established scores have to be measured at the same time in several studies. Each time a relationship is demonstrated, an additional bit of evidence can be attached to the new test. Construct validity is commonly divided into two variants: convergent construct validity and discriminant construct validity. Convergent evidence for validity is obtained if an outcome measure correlates with other tests, which are believed to measure the same construct. Divergent construct validity determines how dissimilar two constructs are, which theoretically should not be related to each other, such as happiness and sadness. Construct validity should be assessed by testing predefined specific hypotheses.[5]

Face validity is the mere appearance that an outcome measure has validity.[2] In contrast to the other variants of validity discussed above, face validity is not a technical form of validity, because it is a subjective appraisement of whether the test "looks like" it is going to measure what it is supposed to measure. Face validity appears to be helpful for the motivation of both the evaluators and test takers, who will be more confident in conducting, and taking, a test if the test appears to be valid.

International Classification of Function

The International Classification of Functioning, Disability and Health (http://www.who.int/classifications/icf/en/) commonly known and abbreviated as ICF and published by the World Health Organization (WHO) in 2001, provides a standard language and framework for the description of health and health-related states independent of specific diseases. Functioning and disability are viewed as a complex interaction between the health condition of the individual and the contextual factors of the environment as well as personal factors.

The ICF is based on a biopsychosocial model and provides a coherent view of different perspectives of health: biological, individual, and social. It is structured around the following broad constructs:

- Body functions and structure
- Activities (related to tasks and actions by an individual) and participation (involvement in a life situation)
- Environmental factors

The ICF has been designed to classify and describe health conditions, and as such it is not an evaluation tool. However, the ICF provides an internationally recognized framework to describe, categorize, and classify outcome measures.

Clinical Initiatives in the Field of Spinal Cord Medicine

Given that presently there are more human SCI studies in progress, or planned, than ever before,[6] a lot has been invested in recent years in outcome measure research in the field of SCI medicine in the form of clinical initiatives and expert panels supported by professional organizations.

International Campaign for Cures of Spinal Cord Injury Paralysis

The International Campaign for Cures of Spinal Cord Injury Paralysis (known as the ICCP; http://campaignforcure.org) is a group of affiliated nonprofit organizations working to fund research into cures for paralysis caused by spinal cord injury. The ICCP developed guidelines, as reported in a series of four open-access publications,[1,7–9] for the design of clinical trials to protect or repair the injured spinal cord. The guidelines for clinical trial outcome measures[1] provide recommendations for neurologic, functional, and quality-of-life assessments to be used in different phases of clinical trials.

Spinal Cord Injury Research Evidence (SCIRE)

The Spinal Cord Injury Research Evidence project (SCIRE; http://www.scireproject.com/)[10] covers a comprehensive set of topics relevant to SCI rehabilitation and community reintegration. The SCIRE project reviews, evaluates, and translates existing research knowledge into a clear and concise format to inform health professionals and other stakeholders of the best rehabilitation practices following SCI. SCIRE provides and maintains the Outcome Measures Toolkit, a list of, currently, 33 outcome measures for use in SCI clinical practice. Comprehensive clinical summaries are available online.

Spinal Cord Outcomes Partnership Endeavor (SCOPE)

The Spinal Cord Outcomes Partnership Endeavor (SCOPE, http://www.scopesci.org) is a broad-based consortium of scientists and clinical researchers whose mission is to enhance the development of human study protocols to accurately assess therapeutic interventions for SCI.[6] Several reports have emerged from this partnership, including the aforementioned ICCP guidelines as well as a review of outcomes measures in SCI,[6] based on a previously developed appraisal framework for evaluating metric properties.[11] SCOPE provides the following regularly updated databases on their Web site (http://www.scope-sci.org/trials.php): Current SCI Clinical Trials of Drug, Cell, and Surgical Interventions to Improve Neurological and Related Functional Outcomes; and Current SCI Clinical Trials of Rehabilitation and Technological Interventions to Improve Functional Outcomes.

International Standards for Neurological Classification of Spinal Cord Injury

The International Standards for Neurological Classification of Spinal Cord Injury (ISNCSCI, pronunciation IN'SKI), published by the American Spinal Injury Association (ASIA), is a widely accepted assessment scheme and clinical communication tool for both clinicians and researchers. ISNCSCI is considered the de-facto standards for describing and quantifying the neurologic deficits caused by a SCI.[12] Sensory function is examined bilaterally in 28 dermatomes for light-touch appreciation (using a cotton tip) and pinprick discrimination (using the rounded and the sharp ends of an opened safety pin). Motor function is tested via a standardized manual muscle test bilaterally on five myotomes (C5–T1) on the arms and five myotomes on the legs (L2–S1). The very important most caudal segments S4–S5 are assessed, in addition to light touch and pinprick, by anorectal examination for deep anal pressure and voluntary anal contraction. ISNCSCI is designed to be a bedside test conducted with the patient in the supine position. No additional equipment is required besides a cotton tip and a safety pin. The time needed for a full examination is estimated as 15 minutes (for complete thoracic lesions) to 60 minutes (for incomplete cervical lesions).

Based on this clinical examination, the SCI-induced impairment is defined by several variables: the neurologic level, the severity (complete versus incomplete and the ASIA Impairment Scale [AIS]), and the zones of partial preservation. The AIS describes the SCI severity on an ascending five-point scale. Grade A denotes a complete injury; grades B to D describe incomplete injuries, and grade E is used only in follow-up assessments to indicate restored spinal function (**Table 2.1**). The zones of partial preservation are used only with complete injuries, and refer to those dermatomes and myotomes caudal to the sensory and motor levels that remain partly innervated.

The ISNCSCI has been an actively developed standard for more than 40 years, currently in its seventh revision, which is available in an updated booklet (http://www.asia-spinalinjury .org/asia_store/asia_store.php). The booklet contains several clarifications and a revised worksheet (**Fig. 2.1**).

The psychometric properties of ISNCSCI are well investigated.[13] Adequate reliability was found in several studies for the total motor score and the sensory scores. Individual myotomes and dermatomes show a more divergent reliability. Substantial to almost perfect Cohen's kappa coefficients (0.649–0.993) are reported for myotomes, and fair to almost perfect coefficients for dermatomes (0.38–1). Children under 4 years of age cannot be reliably assessed with ISNCSCI. Convergent and divergent construct validity was consistently found in numerous previous studies.[13]

Besides measurement error introduced during the examination, classification error also contributes to the overall error. Classification accuracy has been assessed in the framework of formal training sessions, where the attendees rated several ISNCSCI cases before (pretest) and after (posttest) the training.[14] After training, the overall classification accuracy is ~ 90%. The highest misclassifications rates are encountered for motor levels (81.9%) and AIS (88.1%). This error source can be eliminated by computational ISNCSCI classification. Accordingly, several ISNCSCI calculators were developed in

Table 2.1 American Spinal Injury Association (ASIA) Impairment Scale (AIS)

AIS Grade	Definition
A	Complete. No sensory or motor function is preserved in the sacral segments S4-S5.
B	Sensory incomplete. Sensory but not motor function is preserved below the neurologic level and includes the sacral segments S4-S5 (light touch or pinprick at S4-S5 or deep anal pressure) AND no motor function is preserved more than three levels below the motor level on either side of the body.
C	Motor incomplete. Motor function is preserved at the most caudal sacral segments for voluntary anal contraction (VAC) OR the patient meets the criteria for sensory incomplete status (sensory function preserved at the most caudal sacral segments (S4-S5) by LT, PP or DAP), and has some sparing of motor function more than three levels below the ipsilateral motor level on either side of the body. (This includes key or non-key muscle functions to determine motor incomplete status.) For AIS C, less than half of key muscle functions below the single NLI have a muscle grade ≥ 3.
D	Motor incomplete. Motor incomplete status as defined above, with at least half (half or more) of key muscle functions below the single NLI having a muscle grade ≥ 3.
E	Normal. If sensation and motor function as tested with the ISNCSCI are graded as normal in all segments, and the patient had prior deficits, then the AIS grade is E. Someone without an initial SCI does not receive an AIS grade.
Not determinable (ND)	To document the sensory, motor, and NLI levels, use the ASIA Impairment Scale grade or the zone of partial preservation (ZPP) when the levels are unable to be determined based on the examination results.

Abbreviations: DAP, deep anal pressure; ISNCSCI, International Standards for Neurological Classification of Spinal Cord Injury; LT, light touch; NLI, neurological level of injury; PP, pin prick; SCI, spinal cord injury.

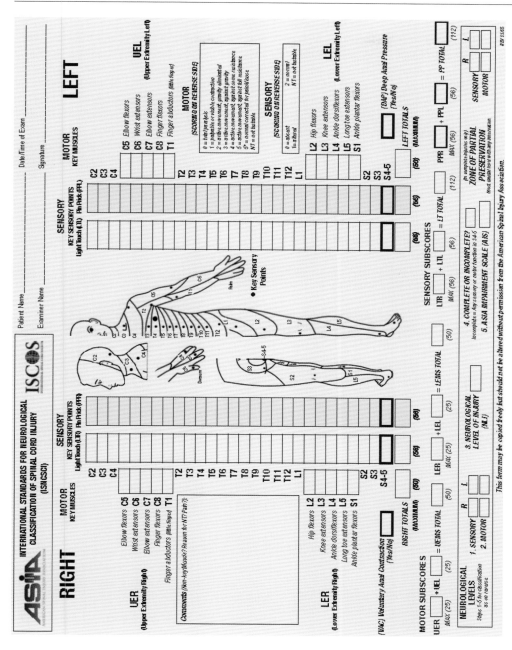

Fig. 2.1 The front side of the current ISNCSCI examination worksheet (revised April 2015). (From American Spinal Injury Association.) http://www.asia-spinalinjury.org/elearning/ISNCSCI.php.)

recent years that generate consistent classifications. Two of them have become widely available online: the EMSCI ISNCSCI calculator (http://ais.emsci.org) and the Rick Hanson Institute ISNCSCI algorithms (http://www.isncscialgorithm.com). Both calculators have been validated on large data sets and produce consistent results for not testable (NT) or missing dermatomes and myotomes using sophisticated logical inference techniques.

Several authors strongly recommend training clinicians in how to conduct a high-quality ISNCSCI examination and classification. Training programs are available online (International Standards Training e-Learning Program [InSTeP]; http://www.ASIAlearningcenter.com) and have been integrated into research networks such as the European Multicenter Study on Human Spinal Cord Injury (EMSCI)[14] and several clinical trials. ISNCSCI is considered a mandatory assessment for scientific journals publishing SCI-related research in which patient characteristics, subgrouping, and neurologic recovery are reported.

Neurologic Function

Many neurologic outcome measures, such as neuroimaging, quantitative sensory testing (QST), and the battery of electrophysiological assessments (e.g., motor evoked potentials [MEPs] and somatosensory evoked potentials [SSEPs]) are constrained in respect to their routine usability in clinical trials. Neuroimaging-based methods, such as magnetic resonance imaging (MRI) and its advanced sequences (e.g., diffusion tensor imaging), require expensive equipment and trained experts to analyze the findings. Moreover, the quality of MRI-based data acquisition may vary considerably due to patient-dependent (e.g., artifacts following osteosynthetic spinal stabilization) and -independent (variability of MRI quality across multicentric sites) factors.

Accordingly, at this point these imaging methods are powerful tools in basic research, but they are not yet applicable to routine clinical trial use. QST represents a sensitive assessment to determine the proprioceptive (dorsal columns) and protopathic (spinothalamic tract) sensory function, but it also requires expensive equipment and training, so that this instrument is more often used in specialized pain or sensory function studies than in general-purpose clinical trials. The same holds true for MEP and SSEP, which provide objective methods to evaluate ascending and descending spinal pathways, but are challenging to establish at multiple clinical sites.

Autonomic Function

Blood pressure and heart rate variability as well as the response to orthostatic challenge (e.g., sit-up and tilt-table maneuvers) are reported to have content validity and reliability, whereas the sympathetic skin response shows only minimal valditiy.[6]

The International Standards to document remaining Autonomic Function after Spinal Cord Injury (ISAFSCI)[15] were developed by an international collaboration between ASIA and the International Spinal Cord Society (ISCoS). ISAFSCI includes two parts: general autonomic function; and lower urinary tract, bowel, and sexual function. The general autonomic function is composed of five items: heart rate, blood pressure, sweating, temperature regulation, and respiratory control. ISAFSCI has been developed as an adjunct to ISNCSCI, and likewise it is accompanied by a web-based training course, the Autonomic Standards Training E Program (ASTeP): http://www.ASIAlearning center.com.

General Functional Status

The Barthel Index (BI), which was developed for stroke, neuromuscular and musculoskeletal disorders, assesses activities of daily living (ADL). The BI consists of 10 items (feeding, bathing, grooming, dressing, bowels, bladder, toilet use, transfers, mobility, and stairs) and has been revised several times, including the development of the Modified Barthel Index

(MBI). In the SCI population, the BI and MBI show floor and ceiling effects as well as inconclusive results in terms of reliability and validity.[16] Therefore, the BI cannot be recommended as an SCI outcome measure. As a consequence the Quadriplegia Index of Function (QIF) was developed for individuals with tetraplegia and introduced in 1980.[17] It is composed of 10 weighted ADL variables (transfers, grooming, bathing, feeding, dressing, wheelchair mobility, bed activities, bladder program, bowel program, and understanding of personal care). The time needed to conduct a full QIF assessment is reported to be less than half an hour. The reliability and validity were reported to be adequate in several studies.[16]

The Functional Independence Measure (FIM) is one of the most frequently used measures to assess basic quality of ADLs in persons with a disability. The FIM is available in several languages, and consists of 18 items on an eight-point scale to assess the amount of assistance the patient needs to perform basic life activities such as self-care, sphincter control, transfers, locomotion, communication, and social cognition. The FIM demonstrated acceptable reliability across a wide range of settings, raters, and patients.[18] For the SCI population, excellent reliabilities and excellent validities have been reported. However, the FIM shows ceiling effects, because the vast majority of individuals with SCI have maximum scores on FIM cognitive items.[11]

The Spinal Cord Independence Measure (SCIM) is now available in its third revision since 2007.[19] The SCIM is the only comprehensive ability rating scale, which was designed specifically for SCI. Three related but distinct domains (self-care, respiration and sphincter management, and mobility) are assessed in 19 items, resulting in a total score between 0 and 100. In-depth psychometric analyses found excellent reliability and validity for the third SCIM version. However, more detailed scoring instructions were recommended to decrease the time needed to conduct this assessment. The time to run the test is estimated to be between 5 minutes (for sedated patients in an intensive care unit) and 45 minutes (for patients with high cervical lesion). The SCIM is validated in several languages, including English, Italian, and Turkish.

Walking, Ambulation, and Balance

Timed tests, for which the only requirements are a stopwatch and a flat, straight, hard surface for walking, include the 10-Meter Walk Test (10MWT), the 6-Minute Walk Test (6MWT), and the Timed Up and Go (TUG) test; these tests are frequently used in the SCI population.[6,20] The 10MWT assesses the time needed to walk 10 m, in order to calculate the short distance walking speed. Different protocol variants have been used. In the recommended variant, a 14-m walkway is used, but only the middle 10 m are timed. The additional 4 m are meant for acceleration and deceleration (to allow for a flying start and stop).

The 6MWT was originally developed to assess the functional capacity or endurance of patients with cardiopulmonary diseases. It measures the distance a patient is able to walk over 6 minutes. Rests are allowed. An even walking course of at least 30 m is recommended.

The TUG was originally developed to assess mobility and balance for elderly individuals. The patient is instructed to stand up from an armchair, walk 3 m, turn around, return to the armchair, and sit down. The time of a full cycle is measured at the individual's preferred speed. Assistive devices are allowed.

These timed measures have excellent intrarater (10MWT: 0.983; 6MWT: 0.981; TUG: 0.979) and interrater (10MWT: 0.974; 6MWT: 0.970; TUG: 0.973) reliability.[21] Excellent validity has been reported in several publications.[20]

In contrast to the timed measures, which can be conducted only in ambulatory individuals, categorical measures offer the opportunity to capture the transition from nonambulatory to ambulatory status.[20] Categorical ambulation measures are provided by the Walking Index of Spinal Cord Injury version 2 (WISCI II) and the mobility items of the SCIM and FIM. The WISCI is a capacity measure of walking function, which categorizes in 21 levels the extent and nature of assistance that persons with SCI require to walk.[22] Level 0, the lowest, indicates the inability to stand or walk with assistance.

Level 20, the highest, indicates the ability to walk 10 m with no devices, no braces, and no physical assistance. Excellent reliability and validity have been reported in several studies. As expected, the WISCI II has ceiling effects for individuals with good walking function who are not dependent on walking aids.

The Spinal Cord Injury Functional Ambulation Inventory (SCI-FAI)[23] has components of a timed test and categorical measures. It has three domains. A gait score indicates the quality of gait, an assistive-device score indicates the use of assistive devices, and a temporal/distance score is the result of a timed 2-minute walk test and a self-reported ambulation classification score. The SCI-FAI is a reliable and valid observational gait score for patients who are already walking, and it takes only a few minutes to administer.

The Spinal Cord Injury Functional Ambulation Profile (SCI-FAP) is another valid and reliable measure of walking skills for individuals with SCI.[24] It includes the timed performance of seven tasks, such as walking and negotiating obstacles, doors, and stairs. By including a daily walking task, it covers the environmental factors of the ICF better than any other validated ambulation assessment in SCI.

The Berg Balance Scale (BBS) is a performance-based measure of balance. Originally developed for use in the elderly, the BBS has been used for various pathologies including SCI. It takes 15 to 20 minutes to conduct a BBS assessment. The BBS is available in several languages, including English, German, Italian, Turkish, Dutch, Korean, and Portuguese. Adequate reliability and excellent validity was reported for the SCI population.[25] However, ceiling effects have been reported for the AIS D subgroup. Moreover the BBS was not able to discriminate between people who fell and people who did not fall.[25]

The motor subscale of the FIM consists of two locomotor-relevant items: walking or wheelchair propulsion (seven-point scale), and stair climbing (seven-point scale). Assistive devices, braces, and walking aids are not considered. To overcome this disadvantage, the SCIM was specifically developed for SCI. The SCIM mobility (indoors and outdoors on an even surface) sub-score consists of six items: mobility indoors (nine-point scale), mobility for moderate distances (nine-point scale), mobility outdoors (nine-point scale), stair management (four-point scale), transfers wheelchair–car (three-point scale), and transfers ground–wheelchair (three-point scale). The resulting subscale total score (0–30) has been shown to have excellent interrater reliability and construct validity.[19]

The combination of WISCI II and 10MWT is recommended as the best-validated measures of walking capacity.[12,20] However, these quick-to-conduct assessments do not cover gait quality, which can be tested with the SCI-FAI. The SCI-FAP is recommended if ADLs need to be addressed.

Upper Extremity Function

There is a general consensus that generic hand function tests are too limited for individuals with tetraplegia and therefore are not appropriate.[26] Accordingly, several SCI-specific assessments for the upper extremities have been developed.

The Capabilities of Upper Extremity (CUE) has two variants. A questionnaire (CUE-Q) and a performance test (CUE-T). The CUE-Q is a measure of functional limitation in tetraplegia, which can be administered by clinicians in interview format. It takes about 30 minutes to complete. The CUE-T is an objective standardized assessment of upper-limb capabilities specifically developed for persons with tetraplegia.[27] The 16 unilateral and two bilateral items were derived from the CUE-Q. It takes 45 to 60 minutes to administer this reliable and valid test.

The Grasp and Release Test (GRT)[28] was specifically developed to assess hand opening and closing and to be used as a functional test with neuroprostheses. GRT assesses the ability to pick up, move, and release six different objects using a palmar or lateral grasp. It takes about 20 minutes to administer. Two studies reported that GRT has excellent reliability and adequate-to-excellent validity.

The Van Lieshout Test–Short Version (VLT-SV) assesses in 10 items the positioning and stabilizing of the arm, hand opening and closing using the tenodesis effect, grasping and releasing of objects, and manipulation of objects using thumb and fingers.[29] It takes 25 to 35 minutes to administer.

The Graded Redefined Assessment of Strength, Sensibility, and Prehension (GRASSP) was specifically developed as an impairment measure for the upper limbs in tetraplegia.[30] It takes 60 to 90 minutes to administer. The GRASSP consists of three subcategories: strength, sensation, and prehension. Strength is assessed by a manual muscle test that extends the five ISNCSCI key muscles test by another five muscles important for hand function. Semmes Weinstein monofilaments are used for testing three palmar and three dorsal key sensory points. Prehension is divided into ability (cylindrical, lateral key, and tip-to-tip pinch grasp) and six performance tasks (pour water from a bottle, open jars, pick up and turn a key, transfer pegs, pick up four coins and place in slot, and screw four nuts onto bolts). A full GRASSP was found to demonstrate reliability and construct and concurrent validity for individuals with tetraplegia.

Pain

Categorizing pain as nociceptive or neuropathic is a prerequisite for providing adequate treatment, and therefore appropriate pain assessment is important. Accordingly, the International Spinal Cord Injury Pain (ISCIP) classification system was developed specifically for SCI by an international group of SCI and pain experts.[31] It consists of three tiers (**Table 2.2**): Tier 1 categorizes the pain type (nociceptive, neuropathic, other, and unknown). Tier 2 documents the pain subtype (nociceptive: musculoskeletal, visceral, other; neuropathic: at level, below level, other). Tier 3 documents the primary pain source or pathology.

The Numerical Rating Scale (NRS) is recommended as a valid outcome measure to assess pain intensity and pain unpleasantness, with fixed anchor labels (intensity: 0 indicates no pain and 10 indicates pain as bad as you can imagine; unpleasantness: 0 indicates no unpleasantness and 10 indicates worst possible unpleasantness). The Leeds Assessment of Neuropathic Symptoms and Signs (LANSS) pain scale discriminates between neuropathic and nociceptive pain. Recently, the Spinal Cord Injury Pain Instrument (SCIPI)[32] has been validated in the SCI population as a new screening tool for neuropathic pain; it takes only a few minutes to administer. Changes in neuropathic pain can be assessed with the Neuropathic Pain Scale (NPS). The International Spinal Cord Injury Basic Pain Dataset (ISCIPDS:B) is designed to

Table 2.2 International Spinal Cord Injury Pain (ISCIP) Classification

Pain Type	Pain Subtype	Example
Nociceptive	Musculoskeletal	Glenohumeral arthritis, lateral epicondylitis, comminuted femur fracture, quadratus lumborum muscle spasm
	Visceral	Myocardial infarction, abdominal pain due to bowel impaction, cholecystitis
	Other	Autonomic dysreflexia headache, migraine headache, surgical skin incision
Neuropathic	At level of SCI	Spinal cord compression, nerve root compression, cauda equine compression
	Below level of SCI	Spinal cord ischemia, spinal cord compression
	Other	Carpal tunnel syndrome, trigeminal neuralgia, diabetic polyneuropathy
Other		Fibromyalgia, complex regional pain syndrome type I, interstitial cystitis, irritable bowel syndrome
Unknown		

contain a minimal amount of the most critical clinically relevant information concerning pain that can be collected in the daily practice of health care professionals with expertise in SCI.[33] The extended version of the International Spinal Cord Injury Basic Pain Dataset (ISCIPDS:E) was primarily developed for research purposes.[33] ISCIPDS contains the aforementioned pain classification system (ISCIP) as well as the NRS for the assessment of pain intensity and pain unpleasantness.

Depression

The 1-year prevalence of depression is three times higher for individuals with SCI (22.2%) than for the general U.S. population.[34] Despite this high prevalence, only a few studies have investigated psychometric properties of depression screening and severity tools in the SCI population. The need for future validity studies cannot be emphasized enough, because most of the depression assessments include both somatic (i.e., neurovegetative) and cognitive-affective symptoms. Somatic symptoms overlap the effects of SCI and will most likely lead to a systematical bias in these tools.[34]

For screening, only the Patient Health Questionnaire-9 (PHQ-9)[35] uses the most current diagnostic criteria for major depressive disorder and has demonstrated adequate accuracy in SCI. PHQ-9 is available in several languages, including English, German, and Spanish, and it takes about 5 minutes to administer in either an interview or self-reported form.

For measuring depression severity, there is even less evidence available for the SCI population, and from the available evidence, it seems that the different measures perform equally well.[6] Therefore, the selection of a particular depression measure cannot be made based on psychometric superiority, but rather on feasibility, acceptability to patients, ease of administration, and the purpose of the evaluation.[6] The Center for Epidemiologic Studies Depression Scale (CES-D) and Beck Depression Inventory (BDI) are the most frequently used measures to assess depression severity, and CES-D has been found to be well suited for epidemiological research.

Quality of Life (QOL)

A recent review found several subjective (individual QOL expectations and achievements) and objective (fulfilling the cultural and societal QOL definitions) QOL outcome measures that have been validated for SCI.[36] The Satisfaction with Life Scale (SWLS) is the most often used subjective QOL measure. It is composed of five items using a seven-point scale, and it takes less than 5 minutes to administer. Several languages are available. The Quality of Life Index–SCI Version (SQL-SCI), which was specifically developed for SCI, has four domains and 37 items scored on a six-point scale and takes about 10 minutes to administer. Construct validity has been established in two publications, but reliability remains uninvestigated. The Life Satisfaction Questionnaires (LISAT-9, LISAT-11) contains nine and 11 items, respectively. Each item is scored on a six-point scale. LISAT takes not more than 5 minutes to administer. Adequate reliability and adequate to excellent construct validity have been reported.[37]

The Short Form 36 (SF-36) health survey represents the most widely used objective QOL measure. It is a generic 36-item, patient-reported survey of patient health. It is composed of eight domains: vitality, physical functioning, bodily pain, general health perceptions, physical role functioning, emotional role functioning, social role functioning, and mental health. SF-36 has been translated into over 50 languages. Internal consistency and reliability are reported to be adequate to excellent in the SCI population, whereas inconclusive results are reported for validity. As SF-36 is not adapted to SCI, some questions may be seen as insensitive to individuals with complete SCI, especially in the acute phase. More research has been recommended to study this instrument in the SCI population.

The Craig Handicap Assessment and Reporting Technique (CHART) has 32 items within six domains. The administration is patient-reported and takes up to 30 minutes. Several studies reported adequate to excellent reliability and validity. Several languages are available, including English, Spanish, and Chinese. A short form (19 items) has been developed, but its psychometric properties have not yet been investigated.

No conclusive clinical guidelines to use a specific QOL assessment are available. Therefore, the choice of appropriate QOL measure should be based on the study objectives and design, as well as on the psychometric properties of the particular measure within the context of SCI.[36]

Assistive Technology

The Quebec User Evaluation of Satisfaction with Assistive Technology (version 2.0) (QUEST 2.0), consisting of an 8-item device domain and a 4-item service domain, is a standardized instrument designed to measure user satisfaction with a broad range of assistive technology devices.[38] QUEST 2.0 must be purchased, and it takes 10 to 15 minutes to administer as either interview based or self-reported. Originally developed in French, several languages are now available, including English, German, Chinese, and Japanese. Reliability and validity studies are available for the Chinese version, reporting excellent internal consistency but only poor to average construct validity.

The Assistive Technology Device Predisposition Assessment (ATD PA) assesses the patient's subjective satisfaction with current achievements in a variety of functional areas. The patient characterizes aspects of his or her functioning, temperament, lifestyle, and views of a particular assistive device.[39] ATD PA has 63 items in two domains and is translated into Italian and French. Excellent reliability and validity have been reported.[39]

Spasticity

The Wartenberg Pendulum Test was introduced in 1950 as a diagnostic tool of spasticity. The clinician drops the patient's foot from a knee fully extended position. The motion and the number of oscillations are measured with a computer. The resulting relaxation index is compared with normative values. This test is not validated in the SCI population. The Spinal Cord Assessment Tool for Spastic reflexes (SCATS) is a validated clinical tool intended to rate spastic motor behavior of the lower extremities after SCI.[40] It consists of three items: clonus, flexor spasms, and extensor spasms. Each item is scored on a four-point scale, rating the reaction to a stimulus as none, mild, moderate, or severe. The combination of SCATS with a self-reported score was recommended. The Penn Spasm Frequency Scale (PSFS) is such a self-reported score covering two items: the frequency (five-point scale) and the severity (three-point scale). No validation studies have been performed for the SCI population.[41]

Singe-joint resistance to passive muscle stretching is rated with the Modified Ashworth Scale (MAS), a widely used six-category ordinal scale. The MAS represents a straightforward bedside assessment. Although the MAS is considered the gold standard of spasticity assessments, only poor reliability has been reported in the SCI population.[42] This is attributable to the fact that it mirrors the tonic rather than the clonic component of spasticity, which is more prevalent in SCI. Here the SCATS might be more sensitive. The MAS shows more reliability in rating spasticity in upper extremities. Employing the MAS in clinical trials should be accompanied by standardization (base position, movement range of motion and velocity) of the examination and training of the examiner.[43]

Due to the multidimensional nature of spasticity, a battery of tests structured along multiple ICF domains was suggested.[6] At the moment a combination of at least two of the aforementioned assessments seems advisable.

Other Assessments

For assessment tools related to other relevant domains that are not covered by this chapter, such as wheeled mobility, sexual function, skin health, community reintegration, colon and rectal function, and other psychological and mental health aspects, the reader should do an online search of ICCP-, SCIRE-, and SCOPE-based resources for further information.

International SCI Data Sets

The ISCoS started a joint initiative together with ASIA to develop the International SCI Data

Sets.[44] As a result of this workshop, guidelines were developed for the recommended minimal number of data elements acting as a lowest common denominator for a common language among SCI centers worldwide. The guidelines should assist centers in developing new SCI databases, and may enable researchers to be more consistent and effective in the design and publication of clinical research studies through the use of standard data elements that enable comparison among SCI populations worldwide. Twenty datasets are available as of August 2015. Some are freely available online (http://www.iscos.org.uk and http://www.asia-spinalinjury.org) without any restrictions. ISNCSCI, ISAFSCI, and ISCIP are among the most advocated International SCI Data Sets and are recommended to be used as outcome measures.

Traumatic Versus Nontraumatic Injuries

Spinal canal stenosis, transverse myelitis, spinal ischemia, disk herniations, tumorous compression, and congenital diseases such as spina bifida can cause nontraumatic SCI. Patients with clinically stable nontraumatic lesions such as one-time spinal cord ischemia have an outcome comparable to that for patients with traumatic SCI.[45] Accordingly, the same outcome measures as described for traumatic SCI can be applied to nontraumatic spinal cord disease. Future studies regarding valid outcome measures for less stable SCIs (e.g., cord compressions) are needed.

clinical communication tool to describe the neurologic SCI level and severity.

This chapter provided a broad overview of available assessments. For the planning of future clinical studies, an in-depth literature search is recommended. The chosen outcome measures not only should be reliable and valid in the SCI population, but also should be suitable for the individual design of the planned study. In particular, the effort required for each assessment should be carefully weighed against the gain of valid informational content.

Recently, more sophisticated psychometric parameters, such as the smallest real difference (SRD), the minimal detectable change (MDC), and the minimal clinically import difference (MCID), have been investigated for outcomes in SCI. In the context of these parameters the clinical relevance of respective assessments can be better determined. For example, the SRD in interventional trials can be clinically interpreted as the threshold that must be exceeded to consider the changed score as "real"[46] (and not due to statistical variance). Ideally, these parameters would be available both for the acute phase after SCI and for the chronic phase, because in the acute phase the high dynamic of natural recovery will lead to other results than in the more stable chronic rehabilitation period. Further studies regarding such clinical interpretable parameters are strongly encouraged. Moreover, clinical trials would greatly benefit from more sensitive outcome measures, which would help to limit sample sizes.

■ Chapter Summary

Valid and reliable outcome measures play an important role in research as well as for clinical purposes. Many resources have been invested in psychometric studies and clinical initiatives, resulting in several well-investigated outcome measures and guidelines that can be recommended. Among the outcomes measures, ISNCSCI is probably the most often used and investigated SCI-specific outcome measure and

Pearls

- Many international initiatives provide guidelines, evidence, and novel tools regarding outcome measures in spinal cord medicine.
- ISNCSCI defines a standardized terminology to clinically describe the neurologic level and severity of SCI.
- Several well-investigated outcomes measures have been established in last decades:
  - General function status: SCIM III
  - Upper extremity: GRASSP
  - Ambulation: 10MWT + WISCI II

with which CSF is obtained in TBI patients through extraventricular drains for intracranial pressure monitoring. Such monitoring is possible, but not typically performed in patients with traumatic SCI, making it more challenging to obtain CSF samples at either single or serial time points.[4] Several CSF biomarkers have been identified with the potential ability of diagnosing acute traumatic SCI, including proteins that indicate structural damage or neuroinflammation. This chapter focuses on markers that have been described in the CSF and blood after acute SCI, and provides a summary of the corresponding studies (**Table 3.1**).

Structural Biomarkers of Spinal Cord Injury in CSF and Serum

Structural proteins that reflect injury to neural tissue are likely choices for biomarkers of injury severity in SCI. Trauma to the spinal cord causes an acute disruption of the spinal cord parenchyma and results in the release of proteins from the nervous tissue into the CSF. Although structural proteins have been studied extensively in TBI and stroke, only a handful of structural protein biomarkers have been investigated as biomarkers in acute SCI.

Glial Fibrillary Acidic Protein

Glial fibrillary acidic protein (GFAP) is an intermediate filament (IF) protein that is expressed in the astroglial skeleton. It is found exclusively in the central nervous system (CNS) and is released from injured glial cells. Evidence suggests it may be a useful marker for various types of brain damage, neurodegenerative disorders, stroke, and severe TBI.[5]

Glial fibrillary acidic protein has been evaluated as a biomarker in a study of traumatic SCI conducted by Kwon et al,[9] in which CSF samples were collected from 27 human patients with complete or incomplete SCI (AIS grade A, B, or C).[9] Intrathecal catheters were inserted for CSF drainage and samples were collected over 72 hours. Kwon et al found that CSF GFAP levels at 24 hours postinjury were dependent on injury severity and were varied significantly in AIS A, B, and C patients. Pouw and colleagues[8]

investigated the CSF-GFAP concentrations within 24 hours of injury in 16 patients with traumatic SCI, and found that the concentration of GFAP in AIS A patients who remained AIS A at follow-up 6 months later was 9.6-fold higher than in AIS A patients who neurologically "converted" to AIS B. More recently, Ahadi et al[6] investigated serum GFAP levels in 35 patients with SCI. Increased concentrations of GFAP were found in SCI patients compared with control patients at 24, 48, and 72 hours postinjury. GFAP levels at 24 hours postinjury were significantly higher in the patients classified as AIS A or B compared with those classified as AIS C or D. Additionally, the 24-hour postinjury levels of GFAP were significantly higher in nonsurvival patients compared with those who survived.

Aside from traumatic SCI, GFAP has been evaluated as a biomarker in ischemic SCI and in TBI. In a study of 39 patients undergoing elective thoracoabdominal aortic aneurysm (TAAA) surgery, GFAP levels in the CSF of patients with and without ischemic complications were compared (reviewed by Yokobori et al[5]). The patients with spinal cord ischemia had significantly higher concentrations of GFAP (571-fold), and the authors concluded that GFAP is a very promising marker for identifying patients at risk for postoperative delayed paraplegia after aortic aneurysm surgery. GFAP has been investigated in many different acute neurologic conditions in both human and animal settings, and appears to be a promising biomarker of injury severity.

Microtubule Associated Protein-2

Microtubule-associated protein-2 (MAP-2) is primarily expressed in the nervous system and is one of the most abundant proteins in the brain.[5] It is important for microtubule stability and neural plasticity, and a potentially useful marker of dendritic injury. MAP-2 has yet to be reported as a biomarker of human SCI, either in the CSF or serum. However, in a rat model of SCI, the extent and time window of MAP-2 loss were evaluated within the spinal cord tissue, and it was found that within 1 to 6 hours after SCI, there is a rapid loss of MAP-2 at the injury site (reviewed by Yokobori et al[5]). Papa et al[10]

Table 3.1 Summary of Studies Describing Potential Biomarkers of Spinal Cord Injury (SCI)

Biomarker	Description	Evidence as a Biomarker in Human SCI	Evidence as a Biomarker in Animal SCI Models	Evidence as a Biomarker in TBI
Alpha-spectrin breakdown products	Generated by the calpain-mediated degradation of submembrane cytoskeletal proteins, namely spectrins	Increased CSF and serum levels in one patient with traumatic SCI[5]	Increased levels of SBDP120 in spinal cord tissue at 6 hpi, and increases in CSF SBDP150 at 4 hpi in a rodent SCI model[5]	Increased in CSF levels in patients with TBI compared with controls; levels were significantly higher in nonsurvival patients (reviewed by Yokobori et al[5])
GFAP	Intermediate filament protein that is expressed in the astroglial skeleton; released from injured glial cells	Increased serum levels in SCI patients compared with controls[6]; Severity dependent expression in CSF from patients with acute SCI[8]; Severity dependent expression in CSF from patients with acute SCI[9]		Increased levels in peripheral blood correlated with unfavorable outcome in patients with moderate-to-severe TBI[7]
MAP-2	Dendritic-specific protein important for microtubule stability and neural plasticity		Rapid loss of MAP-2 at the injury site in a rodent SCI model (reviewed by Yokobori et al[5])	Increased levels in the CSF of patients with severe TBI[10]
NfH	Heavy-chain polypeptide of neurofilament heteropolymer that forms a major cytoskeletal component of axons	Increased serum levels in SCI patients compared with controls[6]; Severity dependent expression in CSF from patients with acute SCI[8]	Increased serum levels in a rodent model of SCI (reviewed by Yokobori et al[5])	Increased CSF levels in pigs after blast-induced traumatic brain injury[11]
NfL	Light-chain polypeptide of neurofilament heteropolymer that forms a major cytoskeletal component of axons	Severity dependent expression in serum from patients with acute SCI[12]		Severity-dependent expression in serum using a rat model of TBI (reviewed by Yokobori et al[5])
NfM	Medium-chain polypeptide of neurofilament heteropolymer that forms a major cytoskeletal component of axons		Increased NfM in spinal cord tissue between 6 and 24 hpi in a rodent model of SCI (reviewed by Yokobori et al[5])	

Biomarker	Description	Human SCI findings	Animal model findings	Outcome / other
NSE	Isozyme of the glycolytic enzyme enolase; localized to the cytoplasm of neurons and usually only elevated following cell injury	Increased serum levels in SCI patients compared with controls[6]	Increased CSF and serum levels in a pig behind-armor blunt-trauma model of SCI (reviewed by Yokobori et al[5])	
S100β	Calcium-binding protein found in astroglial and Schwann cells	Severity dependent expression in CSF from patients with acute SCI[8]	Severity-dependent levels in serum and CSF in a rodent model of SCI (reviewed by Yokobori et al[5])	
		Severity dependent expression in CSF from patients with acute SCI[9]	Increased CSF and serum levels in a pig behind-armor blunt-trauma model of SCI (reviewed by Yokobori et al[5])	
			Increased serum and CSF levels at 6 hpi in a rodent model of SCI (reviewed by Yokobori et al[5])	Increased CSF levels in patients with unfavorable outcomes; levels correlated with intracranial pressure[13]
Tau	Microtubule-binding phosphoprotein highly enriched in axons; released from damaged microtubules due to activation of calpain depolymerization upon injury	Severity dependent expression in CSF from patients with acute SCI[8]	Severity-dependent expression in CSF in a canine model of SCI secondary to intervertebral disk herniation[14]	Increased CSF levels of tau in patients with hydrocephalus[15]
		Severity dependent expression in CSF from patients with acute SCI[9]		
UCH-L1	Highly abundant in the neuronal soma and involved in the addition or removal of ubiquitin from proteins that are destined for metabolism	Increased levels in CSF and serum of one patient with traumatic SCI[5]	Increased levels in CSF at 4 hpi in a rodent model of SCI[5]	Increased serum and CSF levels in patients with severe TBI; UCH-L1 levels were significantly higher and more persistent in nonsurvivors compared with survivors[5]
ILs	A group of cytokines that are involved in the inflammatory process	Severity dependent expression of IL-6 and IL-8 in CSF from patients with acute SCI[9]	Increased expression of IL-1β, and IL-6 in severe, but not mild injury in a rodent model of SCI (reviewed by Kwon et al[2])	

(continued)

Table 3.1 (continued)

Biomarker	Description	Evidence as a Biomarker in Human SCI	Evidence as a Biomarker in Animal SCI Models	Evidence as a Biomarker in TBI
		Increased levels of IL-6 and IL-8 in the CSF of patients with complete SCI (reviewed by Kwon et al[2])		Increases in IL-6 and IL-8 in the CSF and peripheral blood after severe head trauma[16]
MCP-1	A proinflammatory chemokine, involved in the recruitment of type I monocytes; the most potent activator of signal transduction pathways that lead to monocyte transmigration	Severity dependent expression in CSF from patients with acute SCI[9]	Severity-dependent expression in spinal cord in a rodent model of SCI; levels correlated with neuropathic pain (reviewed by Kwon et al[2])	Increased levels of MCP-1 in peripheral blood correlated with unfavorable outcome in patients with moderate-to-severe TBI[7]
MicroRNA	Small noncoding RNAs that are negative regulators of gene expression at the posttranscriptional level		300 miRNA altered in spinal cord tissue following SCI in a rodent model of SCI[17]	52 altered miRNA in serum of patients after severe TBI, with an additional 8 miRNA that are unique to TBI serum[18]
TNF	Proinflammatory cytokine mainly expressed by microglia; plays an important role in the control of cell proliferation, differentiation, and apoptosis	Early elevations in TNF-R1 within CSF of patients with acute SCI[2]	Increased levels in spinal cord tissue after severe, but not mild, injury in a rodent model of SCI (reviewed by Kwon et al[2])	Increased levels in CSF at 24 hpi in patients with brain injury[13]

Abbreviations: CSF, cerebrospinal fluid; GFAP, glial fibrillary acidic protein; hpi, hours postinjury; IL, interleukin; MAP-2, microtubule-associated protein-2; MCP-1, monocyte chemoattractant protein-1; NfH, neurofilament heavy chain; NfL, neurofilament light chain; NfM, neurofilament medium chain; NSE, neuron-specific enolase; SBDP, spectrin breakdown product; TBI, traumatic brain injury; TNF, tumor necrosis factor; UCH-L1, ubiquitin carboxy-terminal hydrolase-L1.

found significant increases in MAP-2 within the CSF of patients with severe TBI. In this study of 152 patients with severe TBI, peak MAP-2 levels within the CSF were higher in patients who did not survive, compared with those who did survive. Thus, it would appear that MAP-2 has potential as a structural biomarker for acute neurotrauma, although studies specifically in acute SCI are lacking.

Neurofilaments

Neurofilaments (Nfs) are a major cytoskeletal component of axons, neuronal soma, and dendrites. The Nf heteropolymer consists of a light chain (NfL), a medium chain (NfM), a heavy chain (NfH), and α-internexin polypeptides. The structure of NfM and NfH includes sidearm domains of differing lengths, and, following trauma, proteolysis of these domains induces compaction of Nfs, resulting in impaired transport and accumulation in disconnected axons.[5]

As a biomarker of traumatic SCI, neurofilaments have been studied in both the CSF and serum. Pouw and colleagues[8] investigated the CSF-NfH concentrations in patients with traumatic SCI, and found elevated levels in patients with motor-complete SCI compared with those with motor-incomplete SCI. Additionally, they found that NfH levels differed significantly between AIS B and AIS C patients. Ahadi et al[6] investigated the phosphorylated form of NfH (p-NfH) in the serum of patients with SCI.[6] Increased concentrations of serum p-NfH were found in SCI patients compared with control patients at 24 and 48 hours postinjury, and levels were higher in patients classified as AIS A, B, or C, compared with those classified as AIS D. Kuhle et al[12] measured serum NfL concentrations in acute SCI patients, who they defined as having either motor-complete paralysis, motor-incomplete paralysis, or central cord syndrome (CCS). Early serum NfL levels were higher in complete and incomplete SCI patients than in healthy controls or CCS patients. Furthermore, the NfL levels increased over time and remained higher in complete SCI patients compared with incomplete and CCS patients. In 2003, Guez et al evaluated NfL concentrations in the CSF of a small series of six patients with SCI and

reported that increased concentrations of NfL correlated with severity of paralysis (reviewed by Yokobori et al[5]). In 2012, Hayakawa et al reported in 14 acute cervical SCI patients that serum NfH levels were elevated as early as 12 hours postinjury, and remained elevated at 21 days postinjury (reviewed by Yokobori et al[5]). The NfH levels in this study were also statistically different in motor-complete patients compared with motor-incomplete patients.

Neurofilaments have also been studied as potential biomarkers in animal models of neurotrauma. Experiments in a rodent model of SCI have reported an upregulation of NfM within spinal cord tissue between 6 and 24 hours postinjury (reviewed by Yokobori et al[5]). In a separate rodent model of SCI, serum NfH levels increased following injury, showing an initial peak at 16 hours postinjury and a second, usually larger peak at 3 days postinjury, returning to baseline levels by 7 days (reviewed by Yokobori et al[5]).

Finally, neurofilaments have been reported as biomarkers in TBI. Recently, a study using a pig model of blast-induced traumatic brain injury identified significantly increased CSF NfH concentrations at 6 hours postinjury compared with preinjury levels.[11] In a rodent model of TBI, serum NfL levels were increased in a severity-dependent fashion, with levels peaking at 24 to 48 hours postinjury (reviewed by Yokobori et al[5]).

Neuron-Specific Enolase

Neuron-specific enolase (NSE) is one of the five isozymes of the glycolytic enzyme enolase. It is localized to the cytoplasm of neurons and is not normally excreted into its environment from intact neurons. Structural damage of neuronal cells causes leakage of NSE into the extracellular compartment, the CSF, and the bloodstream.[5]

Neuron-specific enolase has been evaluated as a biomarker of traumatic and ischemic SCI in human and animal systems. Pouw and colleagues[8] measured CSF NSE concentrations in 16 human patients with traumatic SCI. NSE concentrations were significantly correlated with injury severity (motor complete vs motor incomplete). Ahadi et al[6] investigated serum

NSE levels in 35 patients with SCI. NSE concentrations in the serum were significantly higher at 24 and 48 hours postinjury, compared with control patients.

Several studies were reviewed by Yokobori et al[5]: In a behind-armor blunt trauma model of SCI using pigs, NSE levels were increased in the CSF and serum 3 hours after injury with CSF levels of NSE reaching ~ 3 times that of the serum levels. In a weight-drop contusion rodent model of SCI, serum NSE was significantly higher at 6 hours postinjury, compared with control animals. And in another rodent SCI study of CSF and serum NSE, levels were significantly higher at 2 hours postinjury compared with control, reached peak levels at 6 hours postinjury, and correlated with injury severity. Interestingly, the concentrations of serum NSE were very similar to those that were reported in the CSF.

S100β

The S100 proteins are a family of calcium-binding proteins that help to regulate intracellular calcium. The S100 proteins are found in astroglial and Schwann cells, in addition to adipocytes, chondrocytes, and melanocytes.

Among all neurochemical markers, S100β has been relatively frequently studied as a potential biomarker of traumatic and ischemic SCI in human and animal systems. Kwon et al[9] measured CSF levels of S100β in acute SCI patients and found that 24-hour postinjury concentrations were elevated in an injury severity–dependent fashion. In a separate study of 16 patients with either motor-complete injury (AIS A, B) or motor-incomplete injury (AIS C, D), the mean CSF S100β concentration in motor-complete patients was significantly higher that in motor-incomplete patients.[8]

Two studies were reviewed by Yokobori et al[5]: In a rodent compression model of SCI, Ma et al reported that serum S100β levels rapidly increased following injury, such that by 72 hours postinjury, they had reached concentrations that were nearly five times that of the control animals. And Zhang et al documented an increase in both serum and CSF levels of S100β in a behind-armor blunt trauma model of SCI using pigs; concentrations of S100β in the CSF were reported to be ~10 times higher than the S100β concentrations in the serum.

Aside from traumatic SCI, S100β has been evaluated in TBI and ischemia-induced SCI. In patients with severe TBI, CSF levels of S100β were significantly higher in patients with unfavorable outcomes, and correlated with elevated intracranial pressure.[13] Winnerkvist et al evaluated S100β concentrations in the CSF of 39 patients undergoing TAAA surgery, and found elevated S100β concentrations in five patients who suffered an ischemic SCI, as compared with the S100β levels in those who did not (reviewed by Yokobori et al[5]).

Spectrin Breakdown Products

Spectrin breakdown products (SBDPs) are generated by the calpain-mediated degradation of submembrane cytoskeletal proteins, namely spectrins. The generation of calpain-cleaved degradation products of spectrins has repeatedly been used as a biomarker of various brain pathologies, including those induced by trauma.

Recently, Yokobori et al[5] reported increased levels of SBDP in the CSF and serum of one patient with traumatic SCI, compared with control patients with either hydrocephaly or unruptured aneurysms. In a weight-drop model of rodent SCI, Yokobori et al reported increases in SBDP120 in the spinal cord tissue 6 hours after injury, and SBDP150 in the CSF 4 hours after injury. Yokobori et al reviewed two other studies: In another rodent SCI study, Schumacher et al reported increased levels of SBDP in spinal cord tissue as early as 15 minutes postinjury, with levels peaking at 2 hours postinjury. And in a study of human TBI patients, SBDP levels were measured in serially collected CSF samples taken every 6 hours for 7 days postinjury; SBDP concentrations were increased in patients with TBI compared with control patients at every time point examined, and poor survival was associated with higher SBDP levels.

Tau

Tau is an intracellular protein that is highly enriched in neurons. It is a soluble microtubule binding phosphoprotein and assembles into stable axonal microtubule bundles. Upon injury, activated calpain depolymerizes microtubules. Hyperphosphorylated tau aggregates into filamentous inclusions, termed neurofibrillary tangles that are a strong indication of axonal injury.[5] Tau from damaged microtubules is then released into the CSF and, to some extent, into systemic circulation.

Tau within the CSF has been evaluated as a biomarker of traumatic and ischemic SCI. In a study of traumatic SCI conducted by Kwon et al,[9] tau concentrations in the CSF at 24 hours post-injury were found to be dependent upon injury severity. In fact, in a more recent study by Pouw et al,[8] tau concentrations within 24 hours postinjury were found to be 2.5-fold higher in AIS A patients who remained AIS A at follow-up 6 months later, compared with AIS A patients who neurologically "converted" to an AIS B. In an investigation of 51 dogs with traumatic SCI caused by thoracolumbar or cervical intervertebral disk herniation, CSF tau levels were found to be significantly higher in dogs with lower extremity paralysis as compared with healthy dogs.[14] Furthermore, dogs that improved by one neurologic grade within 1 week had significantly lower tau compared with dogs that needed more time to recover or did not recover.

Tau has also been investigated as a biomarker for traumatic brain injury. The presence of tau in the CSF is a highly sensitive indicator of axonal injury in patients with diffuse axonal brain injury where its levels were shown to increase from 500- to 1000-fold at 1 hour postinjury, to 40,000-fold at 24 hours postinjury and return to normal over the course of a few days.[15]

In summary, tau within CSF has shown promise as a biomarker of injury severity in human and animal traumatic SCI, ischemic SCI, and in TBI.

UCH-L1

Ubiquitin carboxy-terminal hydrolase-L1 (UCH-L1) is highly abundant in the neuronal soma and is involved in the addition or removal of ubiquitin from proteins that are destined for metabolism.[5]

Using a weight-drop model of SCI in rats, Yokobori et al[5] measured an increase in CSF UCH-L1 as early as 4 hours postinjury. Further, in a single human patient with traumatic SCI, Yokobori et al measured increases in both CSF and serum UCH-L1 at 2 days postinjury, with CSF concentrations reaching 50 times the serum UCH-L1 levels. Currently, these preliminary studies are the only existing studies that have investigated the potential of UCH-L1 as a biomarker for acute SCI.

Mondello et al investigated the temporal profile over 7 days of UCH-L1 within the CSF and serum of 95 patients with severe TBI (reviewed by Yokobori et al[5]). They found serum and CSF levels of UCH-L1 to be increased in patients with severe TBI, with CSF levels reaching ~30 times that of the serum levels. The CSF and serum concentrations of UCH-L1 distinguished severe TBI survivors from nonsurvivors, with nonsurvivors having significantly higher and more persistent levels of serum and CSF UCH-L1.

Neuroinflammatory Markers of SCI in CSF and Serum

Inflammation is thought to play a central role in the pathophysiology of secondary injury following acute SCI, and inflammatory mediators such as interleukins and other cytokines may be useful as biomarkers. Cytokines are the central mediators of cell activation and recruitment, and are upregulated at the sites of traumatic injury by resident tissue cells, activated resident and recruited leukocytes, cytokine-activated endothelial cells, and some neurons.

Interleukins

The interleukins are a group of cytokines that are involved in the inflammatory response and can be either pro- or anti-inflammatory, or both, depending on the temporal pattern of expression. Kwon et al[9] found a severity dependent expression of IL-6 and IL-8 in the CSF of human patients with complete or incomplete SCI.[9] In a Taiwanese study of seven patients with acute SCI, an increased concentration of IL-6 and IL-8 was observed in the CSF of patients with complete SCI (reviewed by Kwon et al[2]).

Using a rodent thoracic, weight-drop, contusive model of mild and severe SCI, Yang and colleagues reported that concentrations of the inflammatory proteins, IL-1β, IL-6, and TNF-α mRNA and protein were significantly increased in the spinal cord after a severe, but not mild, injury (reviewed by Kwon et al[2]).

In addition to traumatic SCI, the study of nontraumatic SCI is relevant to the discussion of inflammatory biomarkers. In the CSF of patients with spinal cord injury secondary to transverse myelitis, Kaplin et al demonstrated a 262-fold increase in CSF IL-6 concentrations when compared with control patients (reviewed by Kwon et al[2]). They also found a strong correlation between IL-6 concentrations and the clinical severity of paralysis. In a study of patients undergoing TAAA repair, Kunihara et al found that the occurrence of ischemic paralysis was associated with increased concentrations of IL-8 in the CSF (reviewed by Kwon et al[2]). In patients with severe TBI, CSF levels of IL-1β were significantly higher in patients with unfavorable outcomes,[13] and Kushi et al[16] have found increases in CSF and blood concentrations of IL-6 and IL-8 following severe head injury.

Monocyte Chemoattractant Protein-1

The monocyte chemoattractant protein-1 (MCP-1), also known as the chemokine (C-C motif) ligand 2 (CCL2), is a proinflammatory cytokine that appears to be associated with a poor outcome in studies of brain injury. Overexpression of MCP-1 increases brain infarct volume and exacerbates secondary damage after brain injury, and mouse mutants deficient in genes for MCP-1 show decreased inflammatory infiltration and infarct size.[5]

Kwon et al[9] reported a marked increase in MCP-1 concentrations in the CSF collected from human patients with complete or incomplete SCI, and upregulation was positively correlated with injury severity.[9] In a Taiwanese study of seven patients, an increased concentration MCP-1 was observed in the CSF of patients with complete SCI (reviewed by Kwon et al[2]).

In a rodent model of SCI in which the cord was subjected to impactor forces of 100, 150, or 200 kdyne, there was an increased expression of MCP-1 in the 150-kdyne and 200-kdyne injuries as compared with the mild 100-kdyne injury, and MCP-1 levels correlated with subsequent neuropathic pain (reviewed by Kwon et al[2]).

In addition to SCI, MCP-1 levels in the blood of patients with moderate or severe TBI were increased at admission as well as at 12 hours after admission in patients with unfavorable neurologic outcome, as well as in those patients who died.[7]

Tumor Necrosis Factor

Tumor necrosis factor (TNF) is a proinflammatory cytokine, mainly expressed by microglia, that plays an important role in the control of cell proliferation, differentiation, and apoptosis. TNF recruits macrophages following nerve injury and modulates the expression of cell adhesion molecules, which are required for the migration of leukocytes to sites of injury.

Despite likely playing an important role in secondary injury, TNF has not yet been reported in the CSF or serum of traumatic SCI patients as a potential biomarker. Yang et al reported elevated TNF mRNA and protein in the spinal cord after severe, but not mild injury (reviewed by Kwon et al[2]).

Following human TBI, increases in TNF levels have been reported in both the CSF and serum. Hayakata et al[13] examined CSF from 23 patients with severe TBI and found an increase in CSF TNF concentrations at 24 hours postinjury. The serum concentrations of TNF were over 10-fold lower than in CSF and did not significantly change over time.

Other Potential Biomarker Candidates

Micro RNA

Micro RNAs (miRNAs) are small (18–25 nucleotide), noncoding RNAs that are negative regulators of gene expression at the posttranscriptional level. Microarray analysis has revealed that the expression of over 300 miRNAs is altered following SCI in the adult rat spinal cord.[17] This study suggested that several miRNA (miR-181a, miR-411, miR-99a, miR-34a, miR-30c, miR-384–5p, and miR-30b-5p) target the mRNAs of inflammatory mediators such as intercellular adhesion molecule-1 (ICAM-1), IL-1β, and TNF-α.

Redell et al[18] have investigated the plasma miRNA changes in patients with TBI. Of 108 miRNAs identified in the serum of healthy patients, 52 were altered after severe TBI. An additional eight miRNAs were detected only in the patients with TBI. Further work is needed to determine the utility of these miRNAs as SCI biomarkers.

Classification of Injury Severity and Prediction of Functional Recovery with Biomarkers

Currently, the validation of biomarkers is tied closely to the evaluation of neurologic function using the ISNCSCI standards; however, in time, it is conceivable that biomarkers, by themselves, could provide accurate information about the extent of neurologic injury in patients who cannot be examined reliably. It is well established that the baseline severity of neurologic impairment after SCI is one of the most important predictors of eventual neurologic recovery. Therefore, it would be expected that biomarkers of injury severity would also be able to predict neurologic recovery. After identifying injury-severity–dependent expression of IL-6, IL-8, MCP-1, tau, GFAP, and S100β in the CSF of acute SCI patients, Kwon et al[9] generated a prediction model that used a combination of these markers at a 24-hour postinjury time point to correctly classify baseline AIS grade. Furthermore, these biomarkers were slightly better at predicting segmental motor recovery in cervical SCI than the AIS classification.

Kuhle et al[12] investigated the ability of serum NfL levels to predict neurologic outcome as defined by the mean of the motor and sensory scores at 3, 6 and 12 months postinjury. NfL levels over the first 7 days postinjury were higher in patients with a poor outcome compared with those with a better outcome, with an increasingly stronger correlation over time for NfL measurements after 24 hours.

In addition to the value of having a biological measure of injury severity and objective predictor of outcome, it would be extremely valuable to have biomarkers that could be used as biological surrogate outcome measures in acute SCI. They could then be used to monitor outcome and the effect of interventions. For example, Kwon et al[9] measured CSF NfH concentrations as an indicator of minocycline treatment. Early NfH concentrations (days 1–3) were reduced, suggesting a biological effect on secondary injury mechanisms. In animal models of SCI, it was found that NfH, IL-1β, MMP-9, and NOx were reduced after minocycline treatment, and, in theory, such markers could be evaluated in the CSF or serum of acute SCI patients to document the biological effects of minocycline.[2]

Finally, although the measurement of biological markers within the CSF enjoys the advantage of its proximity to the injured spinal cord, it would obviously be of great utility to establish blood-borne biomarkers of injury. The challenge, of course, is in establishing a serum marker that is specific to the injured process within the CNS and has a sufficient signal-to-noise ratio. For studies that have reported both CSF and blood levels of a given marker, the CSF concentrations are typically much higher, although there are certainly candidates that appear promising in serum (**Table 3.2**). In TBI, several blood-based biomarkers have been investigated; however, examination of only a single molecule associated with damage may lack specificity due to external sources of S100β. Furthermore, systemic inflammatory markers are involved in a vast number of processes, and thus are difficult to individually link to TBI. In the future, a multi-marker approach in characterizing the outcome of acute SCI would be helpful, because the evaluation of multiple markers to establish a "biological signature" could increase diagnostic and prognostic accuracy.

Table 3.2 Studies that Describe Cerebrospinal Fluid (CSF) and Serum Biomarker Concentrations

Study	Indication	Biomarker	"Peak" CSF concentrations	"Peak" Serum concentrations	Comments
Reviewed by Yokobori et al[5]	Rodent model of traumatic SCI with 3 degrees of injury severity	NSE	25.9 ± 3.5 ng/mL	22.9 ± 4.7 ng/mL	Peak concentrations in both CSF and serum occurred at 6 hpi; changes in NSE concentrations in both fluids were comparable and were correlated with injury severity
Reviewed by Yokobori et al[5]	Rodent model of traumatic SCI with 3 degrees of injury severity	S100β	0.84 ± 0.07 ng/mL	0.91 ± 0.12 ng/mL	Peak concentrations in both CSF and serum occurred at 6 hpi; changes in S100β concentrations in both fluids were comparable and were correlated with injury severity
Hayakata et al[13]	Human severe TBI	IL-1β	9.9 ± 1.7 pg/mL	~ 1.0 pg/mL (estimated from figure)	Peak concentrations in CSF occurred at 12 hpi and correlated with poor outcome; serum values were 10× lower and did not correlate
Yokobori et al[5]	Human traumatic SCI	UCH-L1	~ 10.0 ng/mL	~ 0.20 ng/mL	Compared with CSF control and normal serum control in one human patient with SCI, both CSF and serum UCH-L1 levels were increased at 2 dpi
Yokobori et al[5]	Human traumatic SCI	SBDP150	~ 50.0 ng/mL	~ 5.0 ng/mL	Compared with CSF control and normal serum control in one human patient with SCI, CSF and serum SBDP150 levels were increased at 2 dpi
Reviewed by Yokobori et al[5]	High-velocity behind-armor blunt trauma of the spine	NSE	12.514 ng/mL ± 3.096 ng/mL	4.394 ng/mL ± 0.476 ng/mL	Concentrations of neuron-specific enolase were significantly increased in the serum and CSF at 3 hpi, with CSF NSE reaching 3× that of serum NSE
Reviewed by Yokobori et al[5]	High-velocity behind-armor blunt trauma of the spine	S100β	2.585 ng/L ± 1.003 ng/L	0.596 ng/L ± 0.096 ng/mL	Concentrations of S100β were significantly increased in the serum and CSF at 3 hpi, with CSF S100β reaching nearly 4.5× that of serum S100β

Abbreviations: CSF, cerebrospinal fluid; dpi, days postinjury; hpi, hours postinjury; NSE, neuron-specific enolase; SCI, spinal cord injury; SBDP, spectrin breakdown product; TBI, traumatic brain injury; UCH-L1, ubiquitin carboxy-terminal hydrolase-L1.

▦ Future Directions

The challenge of conducting clinical trials in acute SCI that depend on the baseline ISNCSCI examination represents a serious bottleneck in the clinical validation of the ever-growing list of promising therapies. It is in this context that biological markers of injury severity and neurologic recovery may play an important role in the translation of novel therapies. The diagnostic capabilities for the currently available biomarkers cannot exceed that of the initial neurologic assessments, so long as they are compared with these neurologic assessments as the comparative gold standards.[2] However, there is a promising set of biomarkers that may have the ability to stratify injury severity and act as biological indicators of the effects of novel therapeutics for SCI. Future studies are needed to determine whether structural and inflammatory biomarkers could be used as diagnostic markers in those SCI patients where a valid baseline neurologic assessment cannot be obtained, or if they could better predict long-term outcome than this initial neurologic evaluation.

▦ Chapter Summary

The evaluation of biomarkers within the serum and cerebrospinal fluid provides the opportunity to characterize biological mechanisms of injury, monitor injury progression, and potentially predict functional recovery in patients with traumatic spinal cord injury. Currently, clinicians rely on the manual *functional* neurologic assessment, performed according to the ISNCSCI, to identify injury severity in patients. However, in the acute SCI setting it is frequently impossible to conduct this assessment in a valid manner in patients with multiple injuries or brain trauma, or who are intoxicated or sedated pharmacologically. Additionally, even within each ASIA Impairment Scale grade, there is considerable variability in the subsequent spontaneous neurologic recovery of patients with acute SCI. The inability to accurately evaluate injury severity in the acute

setting eliminates patients from clinical trials, whereas the pronounced heterogeneity in recovery necessitates the recruitment of large numbers of patients for acute trials. An objectively measured biomarker of injury severity could increase the number of "recruitable" patients who are eligible for clinical trials and reduce the number of patients required for any one trial. Many efforts have been made to develop potential markers for the diagnosis of CNS disorders. Here, the structural markers glial fibrillary acidic protein (GFAP), microtubule-associated protein-2 (MAP-2), neurofilaments, neuron specific enolase, S100b, spectrin breakdown products, tau, and ubiquitin carboxy-terminal hydrolase L1 (UCH-L1), as well as the inflammatory markers IL-1b, IL-6, IL-8, monocyte chemoattractant protein-1 (MCP-1), and tumor necrosis factor were reviewed for their potential utility in identifying injury severity, and predicting outcome in the preclinical and clinical settings.

Pearls

- ◆ Although the baseline AIS grade of neurologic impairment is used to stratify injury severity after traumatic SCI, its ability to predict outcome is limited, particularly when based on an evaluation early after injury.
- ◆ The cerebrospinal fluid (CSF), due to its proximity to the injured spinal cord parenchyma, can provide insights into pathophysiological responses occurring within the spinal cord.
- ◆ Numerous neurochemical markers have been identified that correlate with injury severity, including inflammatory cytokines, and proteins such as tau, NSE, S100β, and GFAP.
- ◆ The biomarker panel used by Kwon et al[9] was slightly better at predicting the extent of segmental motor recovery in cervical SCI than was the AIS classification.

Pitfalls

- ◆ Although biomarkers within the CSF may provide an objective assessment of the biological extent of injury, they have yet to be validated; at this stage, they certainly cannot be considered a substitute for a thorough clinical examination of neurologic function after acute SCI.
- ◆ There may be a functional "ceiling effect" with the AIS grading system. Conceptually, if the spi-

nal cord is traumatically injured to a degree that produces a functionally complete AIS A injury, doubling the mechanical severity of injury may increase the biological extent of injury, but would still result in the identical injury grading according to the AIS. This may be better represented biologically.
- ◆ As biomarker expression is time dependent, significant variability may be observed when comparing CSF samples obtained from different time points after injury (Pouw et al[8]).

- ◆ Although blood-borne biomarkers of injury would be of great utility, care must be taken due to the lack of CNS specificity of blood. A multi-marker approach could increase diagnostic and prognostic accuracy.
- ◆ The practical implementation steps involved in biomarker development require infrastructural changes for the purpose of storing samples (often in dedicated biobanks) and high-throughput sample analysis technology, as well as careful analysis of variance among different methods, centers, and laboratories.

References
Five Must-Read References

1. Lee RS, Noonan VK, Batke J, et al. Feasibility of patient recruitment into clinical trials of experimental treatments for acute spinal cord injury. J Clin Neurosci 2012;19:1338–1343
2. Kwon BK, Casha S, Hurlbert RJ, Yong VW. Inflammatory and structural biomarkers in acute traumatic spinal cord injury. Clin Chem Lab Med 2011;49:425–433
3. Biomarkers Definitions Working Group. Biomarkers and surrogate endpoints: preferred definitions and conceptual framework. Clin Pharmacol Ther 2001; 69:89–95
4. Kwon BK, Curt A, Belanger LM, et al. Intrathecal pressure monitoring and cerebrospinal fluid drainage in acute spinal cord injury: a prospective randomized trial. J Neurosurg Spine 2009;10:181–193
5. Yokobori S, Zhang Z, Moghieb A, et al. Acute diagnostic biomarkers for spinal cord injury: review of the literature and preliminary research report. World Neurosurg 2015;83:867–878
6. Ahadi R, Khodagholi F, Daneshi A, Vafaei A, Mafi AA, Jorjani M. Diagnostic value of serum levels of GFAP, pNF-H, and NSE compared with clinical findings in severity assessment of human traumatic spinal cord injury. Spine 2015;40:E823–E830
7. Di Battista AP, Buonora JE, Rhind SG, et al. Blood biomarkers in moderate-to-severe traumatic brain injury: potential utility of a multi-marker approach in characterizing outcome. Front Neurol 2015;6:110
8. Pouw MH, Kwon BK, Verbeek MM, et al. Structural biomarkers in the cerebrospinal fluid within 24h after a traumatic spinal cord injury: a descriptive analysis of 16 subjects. Spinal Cord 2014;52:428–433
9. Kwon BK, Stammers AM, Belanger LM, et al. Cerebrospinal fluid inflammatory cytokines and biomarkers of injury severity in acute human spinal cord injury. J Neurotrauma 2010;27:669–682
10. Papa L, Robertson CS, Wang KK, et al. Biomarkers improve clinical outcome predictors of mortality following non-penetrating severe traumatic brain injury. Neurocrit Care 2015;22:52–64
11. Ahmed F, Gyorgy A, Kamnaksh A, et al. Time-dependent changes of protein biomarker levels in the cerebrospinal fluid after blast traumatic brain injury. Electrophoresis 2012;33:3705–3711
12. Kuhle J, Gaiottino J, Leppert D, et al. Serum neurofilament light chain is a biomarker of human spinal cord injury severity and outcome. J Neurol Neurosurg Psychiatry 2015;86:273–279
13. Hayakata T, Shiozaki T, Tasaki O, et al. Changes in CSF S100B and cytokine concentrations in early-phase severe traumatic brain injury. Shock 2004;22:102–107
14. Roerig A, Carlson R, Tipold A, Stein VM. Cerebrospinal fluid tau protein as a biomarker for severity of spinal cord injury in dogs with intervertebral disc herniation. Vet J 2013;197:253–258
15. Cengiz P, Zemlan F, Ellenbogen R, Hawkins D, Zimmerman JJ. Cerebrospinal fluid cleaved-tau protein and 9-hydroxyoctadecadienoic acid concentrations in pediatric patients with hydrocephalus. Pediatr Crit Care Med 2008;9:524–529
16. Kushi H, Saito T, Makino K, Hayashi N. IL-8 is a key mediator of neuroinflammation in severe traumatic brain injuries. Acta Neurochir Suppl (Wien) 2003; 86:347–350
17. Liu NK, Wang XF, Lu QB, Xu XM. Altered microRNA expression following traumatic spinal cord injury. Exp Neurol 2009;219:424–429
18. Redell JB, Moore AN, Ward NH III, Hergenroeder GW, Dash PK. Human traumatic brain injury alters plasma microRNA levels. J Neurotrauma 2010;27:2147–2156

4

Magnetic Resonance Imaging of the Injured Spinal Cord: The Present and the Future

Allan R. Martin, Julien Cohen-Adad, and Michael G. Fehlings

▇ Introduction

Magnetic resonance imaging (MRI) made its debut in the mid-1980s and quickly revolutionized the field of spinal cord imaging, providing unprecedented details of the spinal cord and soft tissue structures, such as disks, ligaments, and paravertebral tissues. Various MRI sequences, such as spin echo, gradient echo, and inversion recovery, have continued to mature over three decades and have achieved reliable, high-resolution imaging that has established MRI as the gold-standard imaging modality for most disorders affecting the spinal cord, including traumatic spinal cord injury (SCI).

However, adoption of MRI into the acute trauma setting has been limited, primarily due to lengthy scan times, challenges with maintaining ventilation and hemodynamic stability in critically ill patients, and concerns about putting obtunded patients in the magnet without performing safety screening. These issues have limited the use of spinal MRI in trauma to a secondary investigation that is often used after initial computed tomography (CT) imaging.[1] In most cases where a neurologic deficit has been identified consistent with a SCI, MRI is indicated to confirm the neurologic level and provide information about the degree of spinal cord compression and structural injury to the ligaments and soft tissues. Most spine surgeons feel this information is essential for surgical decision making, although there is some debate in the community, as some have suggested that the risks of obtaining a preoperative MRI may outweigh the benefits.

Several reports have also suggested that MRI can provide additional prognostic information in acute SCI, by identifying features such as hemorrhage and edema that relate to the amount of tissue damage, and ultimately correlate with neurologic and functional outcomes better than clinical examination alone. However, conventional MRI sequences provide only a macroscopic view of the spinal cord tissue, and signal changes frequently do not correspond with specific pathological processes occurring at the microstructural level, limiting their utility in predicting outcomes. Several new spinal cord MRI techniques are emerging that appear to have the ability to fill this gap, providing quantitative metrics that represent features of the spinal cord microstructure and function.[2] These powerful new MRI techniques have shown tremendous potential in early clinical studies, but it remains to be seen if they can be successfully adopted for clinical use. For now, conventional MRI techniques that provide high-resolution anatomic imaging remain the imaging method of choice for acute SCI.

■ Conventional Magnetic Resonance Imaging in Acute Spinal Cord Injury

The Role of MRI in Trauma Protocols

The efficient management of the acute trauma patient is a complex task that requires a well-organized team to simultaneously stabilize the patient while identifying and prioritizing all severe and potentially life-threatening injuries. These patients are managed according to detailed trauma protocols, evolving over decades of use, to distinguish between patients who require immediate surgical intervention and those who are stable enough to undergo imaging investigations to further characterize injuries in different systems. The choice of imaging modality involves a trade-off between speed and quality of the imaging, and may include a combination of X-rays, CT, and MRI scans. Older trauma protocols relied heavily on X-rays, but modern versions suggest performing only a chest X-ray in the trauma room, followed by complete head-to-tail CT imaging (head, cervical/thoracic/lumbar spine, thorax, abdomen, and pelvis). Cervical spine X-rays, with anteroposterior (AP), lateral, and open mouth views, can also be obtained quickly to identify most cervical fractures, but they have largely been supplanted by CT because they miss 6% of cervical fractures.[3] CT is a highly efficient modality, enabling whole-body scanning in only a few minutes, and has become a cornerstone of trauma care. CT demonstrates the vast majority of spinal injuries, identifies more than 99% of fractures, and demonstrates signs of ligamentous injury (e.g., facet widening) in a majority of cases. CT also provides a degree of visualization of pre- or paravertebral swelling and, to a lesser extent, soft tissues inside the spinal canal suggestive of cord compression. However, to perform CT on a critically ill trauma patient entails ensuring that the patient is hemodynamically stable, setting up portable monitoring equipment, moving the patient, and keeping the patient flat (supine) while in the scanner. All of these steps entail risks to the patient, including the risk of iatrogenic SCI when moving a patient with severe ligamentous injury. Therefore, careful transportation and hemodynamic support are essential to mitigate risk.

Magnetic resonance imaging provides additional information that is complementary to CT, and may have a profound impact on the initial clinical management of SCI patients. This includes the immediate decision making of when (and if) to operate, which approach to take (anterior versus posterior), how many levels require decompression, and what kind of reconstruction is needed. MRI clearly visualizes the spinal cord and surrounding cerebrospinal fluid (CSF), and can demonstrate the degree of spinal cord compression resulting from a fracture, dislocation, disk herniation, intramedullary contusion, or epidural hematoma, any of which could prompt the surgeon to perform decompression with greater urgency. Ligamentous injury can also be identified using MRI, appearing as high signal intensity on certain sequences, which in many cases indicates mechanical instability requiring stabilization with surgical instrumentation (anterior, posterior, or both) and/or external bracing. MRI can also help identify vertebral artery injury (VAI) using MR angiography (MRA), usually performed with injection of gadolinium contrast. Finally, MRI may also be useful for clearance of spine precautions, as it can rule out most spinal injuries, enabling the removal of a hard cervical collar and earlier discharge of the patient. Each of these specific areas in which MRI may affect decision making is discussed in detail below.

Unfortunately, spine MRI protocols typically require a much longer scan time (~ 30 minutes for a standard cervical trauma protocol) than CT—a dramatic increase that may not be acceptable in certain acute trauma patients. All of the risks entailed in performing CT on a critically ill patient, as specified above, are even greater for MRI, due to the increased scan time. If the patient has a concomitant head injury or chest injury, lying supine for this length of time dramatically increases the risk of increased intracranial pressure (ICP) or ventilation problems, respectively. Furthermore, MRI involves a strong magnetic field that requires specialized equipment, which usually means transferring a patient from portable to MRI-compatible monitoring equipment. The magnetic field also poses a serious risk to patients who have surgical implants (pacemakers, aneurysm clips) or metallic fragments (shrapnel, metal shards in eye), and screening for these risks may be impossible if the patient is obtunded or if family is unavailable to provide consent. Thus, the potential benefits of obtaining an MRI must be weighed carefully against the risks.

Both the decision to undertake MRI scanning in acute trauma and the interpretation of the results should be performed by an experienced spinal surgeon, in consultation with the critical care team. It must be remembered that imaging information is simply an adjunct to, and not a replacement for, the clinical information gathered from the history and physical examination. Ideally, a spine surgeon should participate in the initial assessment of the trauma patient to help determine the mechanism of injury and perform a detailed physical examination that includes assessment of neurologic deficits and signs of spinal injury. An examination based on International Standards for Neurological Classification of SCI (ISNCSCI) protocols should be performed once the patient is fully resuscitated and stable. The motor exam may reveal flaccid paralysis below a specific spinal level, a sign of spinal shock associated with severe SCI [American Spinal Injury Association (ASIA) Impairment Scale (AIS) grade A or B]. The patient should be carefully log-rolled to remove the backboard, which can quickly cause pressure ulcers in denervated skin, and the spine should be inspected and palpated at every level from C1 to the sacrum to identify bruising, tenderness, bogginess, and step/gap deformities, which can indicate fractures or ligamentous injuries. Rectal examination for tone, bulbocavernous reflex, sensation (light touch and pinprick at the mucocutaneous junction and deep pressure sensation), and voluntary contraction is an important element of the assessment. The clinical information helps to gauge the likelihood of an injury to the spinal column, and enables an initial CT scan to be interpreted in its appropriate context. The need

to perform an MRI can then be adequately assessed by the spine surgeon, and the scan can be tailored to include only the suspected level(s) of injury and certain sequences, in an effort to minimize scan time.

Specific MRI Sequences for Spine Trauma

Several types of MRI sequences have proven themselves useful for the assessment of traumatic spinal injuries (**Table 4.1**).

T2-Weighted Imaging

In a systematic review of MRI in acute SCI, Bozzo et al[1] found that sagittal T2-weighted (T2W) imaging was used in 100% of studies. This technique provides excellent contrast between the spinal cord and CSF and is the best method to identify the level and specific cause of cord compression, in addition to showing cord edema and intramedullary hemorrhage. T2W is achieved using long repetition time (TR) and long echo time (TE), and is often performed in the spine based on a fast spin echo (FSE) pulse sequence. Sagittal T2W visualizes a lengthy segment of the spinal cord (~ 24 cm) in a small number of slices due to the orientation, and can thus be obtained with a relatively short scan time. Axial T2W is also a useful technique, as it can better identify a lateral disk herniation and visualize asymmetric compression, edema, or hemorrhage affecting the spinal cord. Axial and sagittal T2W can also visualize injury to the facet capsules, seen as high signal, which is particularly sensitive in the lumbar region in the axial plane. However, axial T2W requires a greater number of slices to cover a length of the spinal cord, and thus the scan time can be excessively long. This can be reduced by performing a 3D acquisition or by limiting the coverage to focus only on disk spaces or specifically at the area of injury.

T1-Weighted Imaging

T1-weighted (T1W) imaging is acquired with short TR and TE, and is also commonly performed in trauma protocols.[1] It is useful to

Table 4.1 Conventional and Advanced Spinal Cord Magnetic Resonance Imaging (MRI) Sequences

MRI Sequence (Orientation)	Structures Visualized	Suggested Use
T2W (sagittal)	Cord compression, intramedullary hemorrhage, epidural hemorrhage, edema	Recommended
T2W (axial)	Lateral cord/nerve root compression, hemorrhage, edema	Recommended
T1W (sagittal, axial)	Ligaments, hemorrhage, cysts	Optional
STIR (sagittal, axial)	Ligaments, fractures	Recommended
GRE (sagittal, axial)	Microhemorrhage	Optional
MRA	Vertebral artery injury	Based on Denver criteria
DTI	White matter (axonal integrity, myelination)	Research
MT	White matter (myelination)	Research
MRS	Specific molecules of interest: N-acetyl acetate, creatine, myo-inositol, choline, lactate	Research
MWF	White matter (myelination)	Research
fMRI	Gray matter functional activity, connectivity	Research

Abbreviations: DTI, diffusion tensor imaging; fMRI, functional MRI; GRE, gradient recalled echo; MRA, magnetic resonance angiography; MRS, magnetic resonance spectroscopy; MT, magnetization transfer; MWF, myelin water fraction; STIR, short-tau inversion recovery; T1W, T1-weighted; T2W, T2-weighted.

visualize the spinal ligaments, although this has largely been replaced by the more sensitive short-tau inversion recovery (STIR) sequence. T1W is also complementary to T2W, as the combined knowledge of signal intensity can help identify if a fluid collection is a cyst, hematoma, or fat.

Short-Tau Inversion Recovery

The STIR sequence achieves fat suppression by matching the inversion time (TI) to the T1 parameter of fat, although the suppression is nonspecific and causes signal dropout of other tissues with short T1. The thin spinal ligaments are encased in fat that causes high signal on T1W and T2W, and are best visualized with fat suppression. STIR is highly sensitive for ligamentous injury, appearing as signal hyperintensity, but it should be kept in mind that this technique has limited specificity, tending to overestimate the degree of injury compared with intraoperative findings.[1]

Gradient Echo and Susceptibility Weighted Imaging

Gradient echo (classically termed gradient recalled echo, GRE) and susceptibility weighted imaging (SWI) are techniques that have high sensitivity for identifying hemorrhage, which appears as areas of signal dropout due to the presence of iron in the form of hemoglobin (acute hemorrhage) or hemosiderin (chronic hemorrhage). GRE or SWI may be useful in identifying microhemorrhage within the spinal cord, which has been suggested for the purpose of prognostication, although no studies have reported results to this end.

Assessment of Spinal Cord Compression

In traumatic SCI, the damage to the spinal tissues may or may not result in ongoing spinal cord compression following the initial event. If cord compression is absent following SCI, the urgency to perform surgical decompression and stabilization is substantially decreased. However, ongoing compression is frequently observed due to several causes, which may prompt the surgeon to perform surgical decompression or a closed reduction with greater urgency. In burst fractures, bony fragments are displaced into the spinal canal, decreasing space for the spinal cord and nerve roots. In dislocations such as unilateral or bilateral jumped/perched facets, the canal is narrowed by anterior displacement of the lamina above relative to the vertebral body below. Furthermore, in these cases many surgeons prefer to perform an MRI to rule out a substantial disk herniation prior to performing closed reduction maneuvers, to ensure that the reduction would not cause an increase in cord compression. Herniation or disruption of the intervertebral disk appears in 36% of SCI cases, potentially causing significant cord compression on its own or in conjunction with other factors.[4] The identification of a large disk herniation may also prompt the surgeon to perform an anterior decompressive surgery, such as an anterior cervical diskectomy and fusion (ACDF) prior to, or instead of, a posterior approach. Intramedullary contusions, cord swelling, and epidural hematomas can also reduce space in the canal for viable spinal cord tissue, leading to compressive ischemia. In the context of ongoing spinal cord compression, the notion that "time is spine" is borne out of the same concept as in ischemic stroke, where increased urgency to administer thrombolytic treatments and restore normal perfusion has led to improved outcomes.

Two studies have attempted to directly address this issue in acute SCI. In 1999, Selden et al[5] reported that ongoing cord compression was found in 27 of 55 prospectively enrolled patients (49%), leading to the decision to perform emergency surgery. In a superset of the Selden et al cohort, Papadopoulos et al[6] studied emergency surgical decompression based directly on the results of an immediate MRI scan, and found that the 66 patients undergoing an MRI had improved outcomes compared with the 25 patients who did not undergo an MRI due to contraindications, the need for another emergency surgery, or surgeon preference. In the treatment protocol group, 33 of 66 patients (50%) had an improvement in neurologic status based on the Frankel grade, compared with six of 25 (24%) of the non-protocol cohort. Furthermore, eight of 50 patients (16%) in the protocol group with motor-complete injuries recovered to independent ambulation, whereas none of the 20 patients in the non-protocol group did so. However, these surprising results are subject to several potential sources of bias, as the groups were not randomly assigned and the treatments that each group received were considerably different, partly due to surgeon's discretion. These results suggest that immediate MRI might be highly beneficial to identify ongoing spinal cord compression causing ischemia, supporting an algorithm that many surgeons currently employ in clinical practice.

Identification of Ligamentous Injury

The sensitivity of MRI to detect ligamentous injury is reasonably high: 89% for the supraspinous ligament (SSL), 36 to 100% for the interspinous ligament (ISL), 67% for the ligamentum flavum (LF), 43 to 93% for the posterior longitudinal ligament (PLL), 93% for the disk, and 46 to 71% for the anterior longitudinal ligament (ALL), which adheres to the anterior vertebral bodies.[1] Injuries to the spinal ligaments rarely occur in isolation, and MRI may be useful in localizing and visualizing exactly which ligaments are injured, possibly influencing surgical decisions regarding the need for instrumented reconstruction.

However, MRI tends to overestimate the severity of ligamentous injury, as in the case of a mild ligament sprain that generates edema but not serious damage to the structural integrity, which will show hyperintensity on STIR and T2W. This may lead to excessively conservative management, and many surgeons prefer to rule out clinically meaningful instability with flexion/extension lateral X-rays instead of using MRI.

The Role of MRI in Clearance of the Cervical Spine

In the context of an awake trauma patient without neurologic deficit and a normal cervical spine CT scan (or X-rays), the likelihood of a serious injury is < 1%.[1] In this scenario, clinical spine clearance is appropriate if the patient has no pain, tenderness, and a normal range of motion. If clinical spine clearance fails, then flexion-extension X-rays are likely more useful than MRI, due to their superior specificity for identifying injury; MRI used for this purpose leads to a greater number of patients being discharged with cervical collars.[1] However, in the obtunded patient, an MRI should be obtained within 48 hours to rule out cervical injury and allow collar removal, as per the current guidelines from the American Association of Neurological Surgeons/ Congress of Neurological Surgeons (AANS/CNS). Furthermore, patients with unexplained neurologic deficits should also have an MRI study performed urgently, because CT is inadequate to assess the presence of ongoing cord compression, and timely surgical decompression improves outcomes.

The Role of MRA in Vertebral Artery Injury

Vertebral artery injury (VAI) is an important clinical entity that may cause ischemic or embolic stroke (often including brainstem territory), due to artery occlusion or a thrombogenic dissection, respectively. MRA with gadolinium injection can easily be performed during a trauma MRI protocol, to assess for VAI. MRA may have slightly improved sensitivity and specificity for VAI compared with CT angiography (CTA), due to issues with bony streak artifact that are present in the foramen transversarium and the posterior arch of C1, although no direct comparisons are available using modern 64-detector CT scanners. The

decision to perform imaging studies to rule out VAI should be based on the modified Denver screening criteria for blunt cerebrovascular injury, which include fractures at C1 to C3 through foramen transversarium, or injuries with a subluxation or rotational component. When VAI is identified, the immediate administration of antiplatelet or anticoagulant medication should be strongly considered, while balancing the risk of hemorrhage related to the various injuries that the patient has sustained.

The Value of MRI in Predicting Neurologic and Functional Outcomes

Acute SCI is a devastating condition for patients and their families, and the period following the initial injury is filled with tremendous uncertainty regarding the chances of meaningful recovery. Baseline neurologic status has been established as the most important prognostic factor for final neurologic and functional outcomes, but several groups have attempted to identify features on a baseline MRI that can be used as additional prognostic factors to help improve prediction of outcomes, in an effort to identify the small fraction of patients that make a better-than-expected recovery (**Table 4.2**).

For the purpose of prognostication, most research has focused on the following MRI features: the presence of intramedullary hemorrhage, edema, and cord swelling, and the quantitative measurement of length of hemorrhage, length of edema, maximum canal compromise (MCC), and maximum spinal cord compression (MSCC) (**Figs. 4.1** and **4.2**). Flanders et al[7] investigated cervical SCI patients and found that poor functional recovery was predicted by the presence of intramedullary hemorrhage and the length of edema. The same group reported similar results in a smaller cohort with additional clinical data, confirming these findings, and identified the rostral limit of edema as an additional predictive factor.[8] Selden et al[5] prospectively studied patients with cervical injuries, finding that the presence of intramedullary hematoma, length of hematoma, length of edema, and compression by

Table 4.2 Studies Investigating Independent Prognostic Factors Based on Conventional MRI (Accounting for Baseline Neurologic Status)

Authors (Year)	Study Design; Number of SCI Subjects; Spinal Level	Significant Prognostic MRI Factors Identified	Nonsignificant MRI Features	Comments
Flanders et al (1996)[7]	Retrospective cohort; N = 104; cervical	Intramedullary hemorrhage, length of edema		
Flanders et al (1999)[8]	Retrospective cohort; N = 49; cervical	Intramedullary hemorrhage, length of edema, rostral limit of edema		Cohort overlaps with Flanders et al, 1996[7]
Selden et al (1999)[5]	Retrospective cohort; N = 55; cervical	Intramedullary hemorrhage, length of hemorrhage, length of edema, extra-axial hemorrhage	Length of swelling, maximum diameter of swollen cord, compression due to bone or disk	
Shepard and Bracken (1999)[11]	Prospective cohort; N = 191; all levels	Edema	Hemorrhage, contusion	
Boldin et al (2006)[9]	Prospective cohort; N = 29; cervical	Length of hemorrhage		
Miyanji et al (2007)[10]	Prospective cohort; N = 100; cervical	Intramedullary hemorrhage, cord swelling	Edema, soft tissue injury, preinjury stenosis, disk herniation, MCC, MSCC, lesion length	
Aarabi et al (2011)[13]	Retrospective cohort; N = 42; cervical	Length of lesion, MCC, midsagittal diameter	MSCC	Only included central cord syndrome with preexisting stenosis
Wilson et al (2012)[12]	Prospective cohort; N = 376; all levels		Edema, hemorrhage	MRI signal change used in prediction models with edema = 1 point, hemorrhage = 2 points
Talbott et al (2015)[14]	Retrospective cohort; N = 60; cervical	Extent of T2W signal change on axial section through epicenter		A five-point scoring system (ranging from normal = 0 to most severe = 4); only short-term follow-up (range 4–128 days, mean 23 days)

Abbreviations: MCC, maximum canal compromise; MSCC, maximum spinal cord compression; T2W, T2-weighted.

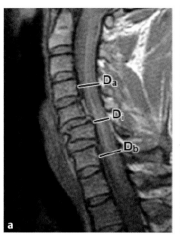 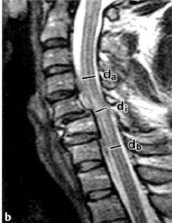 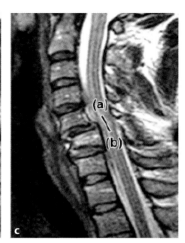

Fig. 4.1 Conventional magnetic resonance imaging (MRI) scans demonstrating maximum canal compromise (MCC) ratio **(a)**, maximum spinal cord compression (MSCC) ratio **(b)**, and length of lesion (LOL) measurements **(c)**. MCC is $2 \times D_i/(D_a + D_b)$, where D_i is the A-P canal diameter at compressed site, D_a is the canal diameter at a normal level above the compression, and D_b is the canal diameter at a normal level below the compression. MSCC is $2 \times d_i/(d_a + d_b)$, where d_i is the A-P spinal cord diameter at compressed site, da is the spinal cord diameter at a normal level above the compression, and d_b is the spinal cord diameter at a normal level below the compression. The length of lesion (LOL) is measured on sagittal imaging from a to b. (Reproduced with permission from Miyanji F, Furlan JC, Aarabi B, Arnold PM, Fehlings MG. Acute cervical traumatic spinal cord injury: MR imaging findings correlated with neurologic outcome—prospective study with 100 consecutive patients. Radiology 2007;243: 820–827.)

extra-axial hematoma were all significant independent negative prognostic factors. Similarly, Boldin et al[9] found that a smaller length of hemorrhage (< 4 mm) showed improved prognosis compared with longer hemorrhage, in cervical SCI.

Miyanji et al[10] reported data in 100 patients with cervical SCI, finding that after controlling for baseline neurologic status, the presence of hemorrhage and cord swelling were both significant independent prognostic factors. In contrast, Shepard and Bracken[11] found that

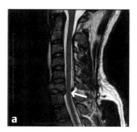 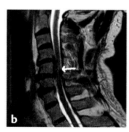 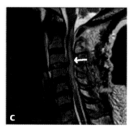 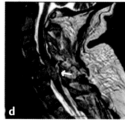

Fig. 4.2 Four patterns of intramedullary signal characteristics *(white arrows)* on sagittal T2-weighted MRI. **(a)** Burst fracture of C6 and retrolisthesis of C6 on C7 by 4 mm with normal cord. **(b)** Single-level hyperintensity indicating edema at the site of severe stenosis (C5–C6) and C5 fracture. **(c)** Multilevel hyperintensity from C1 to C5 indicating edema related to C3–C4 disk herniation. **(d)** Hemorrhage and surrounding edema centered at C6 related to bilateral C5 lamina and inferior facet fractures and anterolisthesis of C5 on C6. (Reproduced with permission from Bozzo A, Marcoux J, Radhakrishna M, Pelletier J, Goulet B. The role of magnetic resonance imaging in the management of acute spinal cord injury. J Neurotrauma 2011;28: 1401–1411.)

Clinical Prediction Rule for Functional Recovery Following Acute SCI

FIM motor 1-year = 50.28 − 0.33 (Age) + 9.17 (AIS grade) − 4.83 (MRI signal)

Probability of functional independence at 1 year =

$$\frac{\exp[-2.93 - 0.03(\text{Age}) + 1.35(\text{AMS}) + 1.36(\text{AIS grade}) - 0.29(\text{MRI signal})]}{(1 + \exp[2.93 - 0.03(\text{Age}) + 1.35(\text{AMS}) + 1.36(\text{AIS grade}) - 0.29(\text{MRI signal})]}$$

Where:
FIM is the Functional Independence Measure.
Age: continuous variable > 16.
AMS: ASIA motor score ≤ 50; ASIA motor score > 50 = 1; < 50 = 0.
AIS grade: AIS grade A= 1; AIS grade B = 2; AIS grade C = 3; AIS grade D = 4.
MRI Signal: No signal change = 0; Sign. cons. w/ edema = 1, Signal consistent with hemorrhage = 2; EXP: Natural logarithm.

Source: From Wilson JR, Grossman RG, Frankowski RF, et al. A clinical prediction model for long-term functional outcome after traumatic spinal cord injury based on acute clinical and imaging factors. J Neurotrauma 2012;29:2263–2271. Reprinted by permission.

---

hemorrhage did not correlate with severity of injury or offer useful prognostic information, after correcting for baseline neurologic status; they analyzed retrospective data in cervical and thoracic SCI patients among the National Acute Spinal Cord Injury Study-3 (NASCIS 3) cohort who had an elective MRI within 72 hours of injury. Furthermore, Wilson et al[12] reported that the presence of T2W signal change (edema or hemorrhage) was not a statistically significant independent predictor of functional outcome in two clinical prediction models that were based on prospective registry data from 376 patients (p = 0.19 and p = 0.54, respectively) **(see text box)**.

The first model used linear regression to predict the functional independence measure (FIM) score at 1 year, including baseline neurologic status, age, and MRI signal characteristics (1 point for edema or 2 points for hemorrhage), and showed moderately strong predictive results (R^2 = 0.52). A second logistic model was also created to predict the probability of logistic independence at 1-year, based on

the same independent variables. Aarabi et al[13] focused specifically on patients with a motor-incomplete lesion consistent with central cord syndrome, finding that none of these patients had macroscopic hemorrhage on MRI. In this group, the length of lesion, MCC, and midsagittal diameter of the spinal cord at the level of MCC were all independently predictive of outcome, whereas the measure of MSCC was not. Most recently, a novel approach was employed by Talbott et al,[14] assessing T2 signal change in an axial cross section of the spinal cord through the injury epicenter. The method uses a four-point scale ranging from 0 for a normal axial image to 4 for whole-cord edema with signs of hemorrhage (**Fig. 4.3**), and results in 60 patients with cervical injury show a strong correlation (R = −0.88) with the AIS grade at hospital discharge (mean 23 days postinjury). However, these results need to be validated with long-term follow-up data and a complete analysis that calculates the independent predictive power of this scoring system.

Considering the overall body of evidence, it appears that the MRI features of edema and hemorrhage likely have weak to moderate utility in helping to predict outcomes, as adjuncts to the primary predictor of baseline neurologic status. However, further research is needed to clarify the value of these prognostic measures, as the current literature contains substantial heterogeneity in terms of methodology and results. The mixed results regarding the prognostic value of MRI in acute SCI highlight the fact that conventional MRI provides little information regarding the health and integrity of the spinal cord tissue itself. MRI features, such as intramedullary hemorrhage and edema, are poor surrogates for the amount of damage to the white matter (WM), gray matter (GM), and myelin. If these characteristics of injury could be accurately determined via imaging, MRI could possibly surpass baseline neurologic status as the most important predictor of outcomes. Furthermore, signal intensity changes labeled as "edema" are in fact nonspecific, and more accurately reflect a multitude of pathophysiological processes that are occurring related to secondary injury mechanisms. Thus, features based on conventional MRI are ultimately of

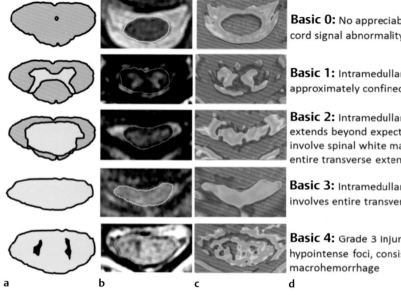

Basic 0: No appreciable intramedullary cord signal abnormality

Basic 1: Intramedullary T2 hyperintensity is approximately confined to central gray matter

Basic 2: Intramedullary T2 hyperintensity extends beyond expected gray matter margins to involve spinal white matter, but does not involve entire transverse extent of the spinal cord

Basic 3: Intramedullary T2 hyperintensity involves entire transverse extent of spinal cord

Basic 4: Grade 3 injury plus discrete T2 hypointense foci, consistent with macrohemorrhage

a   b   c   d

Fig. 4.3 Description of a rating scale using a single axial T2-weighted image through the injury epicenter for prognosis, ranging from 0 (normal) to 4 (most severe). **(a)** Schematics for each rating level. **(b)** Representative axial T2-weighted MRI images. **(c)** Three-dimensional color surface plots based on T2-weighted signal. **(d)** Definitions of each rating level. (Reproduced with permission from Talbott JF, Whetstone WD, Readdy WJ, et al. The Brain and Spinal Injury Center score: a novel, simple, and reproducible method for assessing the severity of acute cervical spinal cord injury with axial T2-weighted MRI findings. J Neurosurg Spine 2015;23:495–504.)

somewhat limited value in prognostication, and it is unlikely that future research focusing on hemorrhage, edema, and cord compression would add substantially to this field. Better imaging tools are needed that more accurately reflect the integrity of the WM and GM within the spinal cord.

▓ The Future of Spinal Cord Imaging

Advanced MRI Techniques

A 2013 meeting of international leaders in the spinal cord imaging community, invited by the International Spinal Research Trust (ISRT) and the Wings for Life (WfL) Spinal Cord Research Foundation, outlined five advanced MRI techniques that have the potential to revolutionize the field by elucidating details of the microstructure and functional organization within the spinal cord (the last five entries in **Table 4.1**).[2] This group highlighted the following techniques due to their ability to characterize microstructural features of the spinal cord: diffusion tensor imaging (DTI), magnetization transfer (MT), myelin water fraction (MWF), and magnetic resonance spectroscopy (MRS). DTI measures the directional diffusivity of water, and several of the metrics that it produces correlate with axonal integrity. MT involves an off-resonance saturating prepulse that takes advantage of the relationship between lipid macromolecules, such as myelin, and nearby water protons, and provides a surrogate measure of myelin quantity. This is most often expressed in a ratio, usually between scans with and without the pre-pulse (MTR), or between the spinal cord and cerebrospinal fluid (MTCSF). MWF measures the quantity of myelin more directly, based on T2 relaxation that uses a multiecho sequence to estimate the T2 parameter in each compartment (myelin, tissue, and CSF). MRS quantifies either the absolute or relative concentrations of specific molecules of interest within a single large voxel, most commonly including N-acetylaspartate (NAA), myo-inositol (Ins), choline (Cho), creatine (Cre), and lactate (Lac). In addition, the expert panel highlighted functional MRI (fMRI) of the spinal cord, due to its potential to characterize changes in neurologic function, based on the blood-oxygen level dependent (BOLD) signal change, which relies on the concept of neurovascular coupling in which changes in neurologic function produce corresponding changes in local blood flow. fMRI studies can involve a variety of designs, including motor tasks or sensory stimuli in block or event-related designs, and can visualize and provide indirect measures reflecting neuronal activity and connectivity directly in the spinal cord.

All five of these emerging MRI techniques are highly amenable to quantitative analysis, setting them apart from conventional MRI and offering the opportunity to develop quantitative MRI biomarkers that correlate with neurologic and functional impairment and reflect specific aberrant processes within the cord tissue. Furthermore, quantitative biomarkers could act as surrogate outcome measures in clinical trials, which could provide short-term end points and reduce the time and costs associated with novel drug development. These techniques could also potentially discriminate reversible and irreversible components of damage (demyelination, axonal loss, gray matter loss) early after injury, and thus provide a more accurate prognosis to help guide therapeutic strategies and focus rehabilitation resources.

Unfortunately, the application of these advanced MRI techniques to imaging the spinal cord is far from trivial. These techniques were initially developed and validated in brain imaging, but the spinal cord is a far more challenging structure in which to obtain accurate data. In fact, the spine is among the most hostile environments in the body for MRI, due to magnetic field inhomogeneity at the interfaces among bone, intervertebral disk, and CSF, and due to the relatively large motion of the cord during cardiac and respiratory cycles.[2] High-quality spinal cord imaging using these methods has only recently been achieved, often requiring specialized acquisition sequences,

complex shimming, custom receive coils, long acquisition times, and substantial postprocessing to correct for motion, aliasing, and other artifacts.

Current Body of Evidence

To date, only a small number of studies have employed these new techniques in the context of spinal cord injury, and none has reported the prediction of neurologic or functional outcomes in a longitudinal study design (**Table 4.3**). In 2004, Stroman et al[15] demonstrated the feasibility of fMRI of the lumbosacral spinal cord below the level of injury in 27 chronic SCI (cSCI) patients, finding that spinal cord activation in response to thermal stimulation was less focused in the ipsilateral dorsal horn compared with healthy subjects. Cadotte et al[16] employed similar techniques in the cervical cord, finding that 18 cSCI subjects had an increase in the number of active voxels with stimulation above the level of injury, and this number correlated with the degree of sensory impairment in abnormal dermatomes.

In contrast, several other groups have employed DTI to image the integrity of the WM, in both the acute SCI (aSCI)[17–19] and cSCI populations.[20–23] Shanmuganathan et al[18] found that in 20 patients in the acute phase of SCI, mean diffusivity (MD) and the primary eigenvector are both decreased in magnitude at the site of injury and rostral to the injury. Cheran et al[17] confirmed these findings in 25 patients, showing that MD, fractional anisotropy (FA), and axial diffusivity (AD) were all decreased. This study also found that in the nonhemorrhagic subgroup, strong correlations were present between DTI metrics and baseline ASIA motor score, suggesting that DTI can accurately assess the degree of tissue injury. More recently, Vedantam et al[19] studied 12 aSCI patients and found that FA at C1–C2, rostral to the site of injury, was significantly decreased compared with healthy controls. These authors also extracted the FA value in the lateral corticospinal tracts (LCSTs), finding moderate to strong correlations with AIS (Spearman $r = 0.71$) and upper limb motor score ($r = 0.67$). In the cSCI population ($N = 18$), Kamble et al[21] also found decreased FA above and below the lesion, compared with healthy

Table 4.3 State-of-the-Art MRI Techniques in Spinal Cord Injury (SCI)

Authors (Year)	Advanced MRI Technique	Study Population	Anatomic Region; Slice Prescription	MRI Acquisition Details
Stroman et al (2004)[15]	fMRI	cSCI (N = 27) and healthy subjects (N = 15)	Lumbar cord; 5 axial slices (mid-disk or mid-VB)	• Single-shot FSE, PD-weighted, SEEP contrast • FOV = 120 × 120 mm^2; matrix = 128 × 128; resolution = 0.9 × 0.9 × ? mm^3; TR/TE = 8,250/34 • Temporal resolution = 8.25 s/volume • Block design, thermal stimulus (10°C, 32°C) to leg dermatomes
Shanmuganathan et al (2008)[18]	DTI	aSCI (N = 20) and healthy subjects (N = 8)	Cervical cord; 67 axial slices, contiguous	• Single-shot EPI, partial Fourier readout, GRAPPA parallel factor = 2 • 6 directions, b = 1,000 second mm^2 • FOV = 200 × 200 mm^2; matrix = 128 × 128; resolution = 1.6 × 1.6 × 3 mm^3; TR/TE = 8,000/76
Cheran et al (2011)[17]	DTI	aSCI (N = 25) and healthy subjects (N = 11)	Cervical cord; 67 axial slices, contiguous	• Same as Shanmuganathan et al (2008)[18]
Cohen-Adad et al (2011)[20]	DTI, MT	cSCI (N = 14) and healthy subjects (N = 14)	Cervical cord; DTI: 8 axial slices, mid-VB, MT: 52 axial slices, 0.4-mm gap	DTI: • Single-shot EPI, GRAPPA parallel factor = 2 • 64 directions, b = 1,000 second mm^2 • FOV = 128 × 128 mm^2; matrix = 128 × 128; resolution = 1 × 1 × 5 mm^3; TR/TE = 1 heartbeat/76 (cardiac gated) • Acquisition repeated × 4 (averaged offline) MT: • 3D gradient echo ± MT pre-pulse (gaussian shape, 1.2kHz offset, 10-ms duration) • FOV = 230 × 230 mm^2; matrix = 256 × 256; resolution = 0.9 × 0.9 × 2 mm^3; TR/TE = 28/3.2
Kamble et al (2011)[21]	DTI	cSCI (N = 18) and healthy subjects (N = 11)	Cervical or lumbar cord; axial slices, contiguous	• EPI • 25 directions, b = 1,000 second mm^2 • FOV = 260 × 260 mm^2; matrix = 128 × 128; resolution = 2 × 2 × 5 mm^3; TR/TE = 8,500/98

Analysis Methods	Clinical Data Reported	Major Results
Activation maps created for L1-S1 spinal cord, individuals co-registered with anatomic template, group activations include voxels active in ≥ 3 subjects	• AIS grade	• Active voxels found in lumbar cord in all cSCI subjects • Complete SCI subjects showed decreased ipsilateral dorsal activation and increased bilateral ventral activation (statistical significance not calculated)
DTI metrics calculated: FA, MD, RA, VR, λ_1, λ_2, λ_3; 3 manual ROIs drawn to include GM and WM at upper, middle, and lower cervical levels	• None	• Decreased MD versus HCs in all 3 ROIs: $p \le 0.01$ • Decreased λ_1 versus HCs in all 3 ROIs: $p \le 0.002$
DTI metrics calculated: FA, MD, AD, RD; 3 manual ROIs drawn on midsagittal reconstructed slice at upper, middle, and lower cervical levels (avoiding hemorrhage)	• ASIA motor score • FU data in 12 subjects (at 1–29 months)	• FA reduced at C3–C5, C6–T1 (NHC: $p < 0.001$, HC: $p < 0.05$) and at injury site ($p < 0.001$) • MD, AD reduced in all regions ($p < 0.001$) • All metrics correlated with motor score in NHC ($R = 0.78$–0.92)
DTI metrics calculated: FA, MD, AD, RD, GFA; MT metrics calculated: MTR; 4 manual ROIs drawn in each axial slice, in the ACs, DCs, and left/right LCSTs (levels with T2W lesion were skipped)	• ASIA motor and sensory scores	• Decreased FA, GFA ($p < 0.0001$) and AD, RD ($p = 0.01$) • FA, GFA, RD correlate with total ASIA (abs $r = 0.66$–0.74, $p < 0.01$) • Tract-specific metrics: weak specificity with motor versus sensory scores • Decreased MTR: 26 versus 32, $p < 0.0001$ • MTR correlates with total ASIA score: $r = 0.59$, $p = 0.04$ • MTR of ACs/LCs more specifically predicts motor score ($p = 0.03$), dorsal region predicts sensory score ($p = 0.03$)
DTI metrics calculated: FA; 3 manual ROIs positioned randomly	• None	• FA in areas above/below lesion decreased versus HCs: 0.37 versus 0.55, $p = 0.001$

(*continued*)

Table 4.3 (*continued*)

Authors (Year)	Advanced MRI Technique	Study Population	Anatomic Region; Slice Prescription	MRI Acquisition Details
Cadotte et al (2012)[16]	fMRI	cSCI (N = 18) and healthy subjects (N = 20)	Cervical cord; 9 sagittal slices, contiguous	• Single-shot FSE, partial Fourier (HASTE), multi-echo, PD-weighted, SEEP contrast • FOV = 280 × 210 mm^2; matrix = 192 × 144; resolution = 1.5 × 1.5 × 2 mm^3; TR/TE = 9,000/38 • Temporal resolution = 9 s/ volume • Thermal (44°C) stimulus, left and right sides in cervical dermatomes above and below injury
Peterson et al (2012)[23]	DTI	cSCI (N = 19) and healthy subjects (N = 28)	Regions at C3-C4, T5, and T12; 6 axial slices per region, contiguous	• Reduced FOV, single-shot EPI, partial Fourier, NEX = 12 • Number of directions NR, b = 750 second mm^2 • FOV = 120 × 30 mm^2; matrix = 176 × 44; resolution = 0.7 × 0.7 × 5 mm^3; TR/TE = 4,000/49; acquisition time = 30 m for 3 regions
Koskinen et al (2013)[22]	DTI	cSCI (N = 28) and healthy subjects (N = 40)	Cervical cord; axial slices, 1.2-mm gap	• EPI, NEX = 4 • 20 directions, b = 1,000 second mm^2 • FOV = 152 × 152 mm^2; matrix = 128 × 128; resolution = 1.2 × 1.2 × 4 mm^3; TR/TE = 4,000/103
Vedantam et al (2015)[19]	DTI	aSCI (N = 12) and healthy subjects (N = 12)	Cervical cord	• Pulse sequence NR • 15 or 25 directions, b = 500 or 600 second mm^2 • FOV = 190 × 190 mm^2; matrix = 128 × 128; resolution = 1.5 × 1.5 ×? mm^3; TR/TE = 5,000/98

Abbreviations: AD, axial diffusivity; AIS, American Spinal Injury Association Impairment Scale; aSCI, acute spinal cord injury; ASIA, American Spinal Injury Association; cSCI, chronic spinal cord injury; DC, dorsal column; DTI, diffusion tensor imaging; EPI, echo planar imaging; FA, fractional anisotropy; FIM, functional independence measure; fMRI, functional MRI; FOV, field of view; FSE, fast spin echo; FU, follow-up; GFA, generalized fractional anisotropy; GLM, general linear model; GM, gray matter; GRAPPA, generalized autocalibrating partial parallel acquisition; HASTE, half fourier acquisition single-shot turbo spin echo; HC, healthy control; LC, lateral column; LCST, lateral corticospinal tract; MD, mean diffusivity; MEP, motor evoked potential; MT, magnetization transfer; MTR, magnetization transfer ratio; NEX, number of excitations; NHC, non-hemorrhagic contusions; NR, not reported; PD, proton density; RA, relative anisotropy; RD, radial diffusivity; ROI, region of interest; SEEP, signal enhancement by extravascular protons; SNR, signal-to-noise ratio; SSEP, somatosensory evoked potential; T2W, T2-weighted; VB, vertebral body; VC, ventral column; VR, volume ratio; WM, white matter.

Analysis Methods	Clinical Data Reported	Major Results
Data analyzed with GLM, normalized and averaged for group activations; clusters of $\geq$ 5 active voxels (positive or negative) analyzed; number of active voxels recorded in each cord quadrant; connectivity analysis performed using coactivations	• ASIA sensory score	• Increased number of active voxels in incomplete cSCI in dermatome of normal sensation • Number of active voxels correlates with degree of sensory impairment: $R^2 = 0.93$, $p < 0.001$ • Increased number of intraspinal connections in cSCI versus HCs
DTI metrics calculated: FA, MD; 5 manual ROIs drawn on each slice (slices with SNR < 20 excluded): whole-cord, left/right LCSTs and left/right DCs	• AIS • SSEPs • MEPs	• FA (C2) decreased in whole-cord, LCSTs, and DCs ($p < 0.005$) • FA (C2) correlates with AIS in each ROI: whole-cord ($r = 0.64$, $p = 0.001$), LCSTs ($r = 0.50$, $p = 0.002$), and DCs ($r = 0.41$, $p = 0.01$) • Mean FA of DCs correlates with tibial SSEP amplitude ($r = 0.46$, $p < 0.001$)
DTI metrics calculated: FA, MD, AD, RD; 2 manual ROIs drawn in, whole-cord at C2-C3 and the rostral edge of lesion	• ASIA • FIM	• Decreased FA at C2-C3: 0.58 versus 0.69, $p < 0.001$ • Increased MD and RD at C2-C3: $p < 0.001$ • FA, MD significantly altered at lesion level ($p < 0.001$) • FA at lesion correlates with ASIA motor: $r = 0.67$, $p < 0.01$
DTI metrics calculated: FA; 2 manual ROIs drawn for whole-cord and bilateral LCSTs at C1-C2	• ASIA motor, sensory scores • AIS	• FA decreased at C1-C2 in whole-cord (0.61 versus 0.67, $p < 0.01$) and LCSTs (0.66 versus 0.70, $p = 0.04$) • FA of LCSTs correlates with AIS ($r = 0.71$, $p = 0.01$), and upper limb motor score ($r = 0.67$, $p = 0.01$) • DTI metrics did not correlate with sensory scores

controls. Petersen et al[23] confirmed the finding of decreased FA rostral to the injury site in 19 cSCI patients, and found correlations between whole-cord FA and AIS (r = 0.64) and between FA of the dorsal columns (DCs) and tibial nerve somatosensory evoked potentials (SSEPs) (r = 0.46). Koskinen et al[22] also found decreased FA above the level of injury in 28 cSCI patients, in addition to increased MD and radial diffusivity (RD). This group also found significant changes in FA and MD at the lesion level, and FA at the lesion correlated well with ASIA motor score (r = 0.67). Cohen-Adad et al[20] utilized the technique of MT in combination with DTI to study 14 cSCI patients, finding highly significant changes in terms of decreased FA and AD, and increased RD compared with healthy subjects. Tract-specific metrics also correlated well with overall ASIA motor and sensory scores, although there was poor specificity of these changes relating FA in the LCSTs and DCs to corresponding motor and sensory subscores, respectively.

Future Directions

Looking ahead, longitudinal studies are needed that apply these powerful new techniques to the aSCI population to determine if they can provide useful prognostic information. Unfortunately, it is difficult and costly to implement such studies, as strong technical expertise is needed and patient recruitment in the acute stage of SCI remains extremely challenging. Furthermore, these acquisition techniques continue to evolve as new discoveries and refinements are made, creating the problem that a specific imaging protocol could be rendered obsolete by the time a longitudinal study is completed. However, the potential benefits to SCI patients of improved diagnostics and prognostication are profound, providing a strong impetus for researchers to take on the challenge of clinical translation of these advanced techniques.

Chapter Summary

Magnetic resonance imaging is a powerful tool for imaging the spinal cord, and can provide important information that may influence immediate decision making and improve prognostication in acute SCI. If ongoing spinal cord compression is identified by MRI, immediate decompression through closed reduction or surgical decompression is indicated to improve outcomes. Ligamentous injury can be detected on MRI that may influence the decision to perform surgical reconstruction. In addition, MRA can identify VAI, which usually prompts antiplatelet or anticoagulant administration. A baseline MRI can also provide information that may improve prognostication, such as the presence and length of intramedullary hemorrhage, the presence and length of edema, the rostral limit of edema, cord swelling, and the degree of cord compression. Unfortunately, all of these MRI features appear to offer only weak prognostic factors, and should be used in conjunction with baseline neurologic status. There are substantial risks associated with obtaining an MRI in a critically ill trauma patient, which the spine surgeon and critical care team must weigh carefully against the potential benefits. Future studies are needed to clarify the optimal role of conventional MRI for immediate decision making and better define the value of conventional and advanced MRI techniques for prognostication. Several emerging spinal cord imaging techniques are likely to dramatically expand our ability to quantify injury, which has important implications for clinical management and research into all pathologies affecting the spinal cord.

results in unbalanced parasympathetic supply associated with vasodilation, bradycardia, and hypotension. This phenomenon is known as neurogenic shock. Note that neurogenic shock is distinct from spinal shock, which also accompanies an acute SCI and reflects loss of reflexes below the level injured. Neurogenic shock is best managed with initial fluid resuscitation, but caution is needed as these patients are easily fluid overloaded. Early consideration should be given to vasopressors with both α- and β-adrenergic activity such as epinephrine and norepinephrine, which increase vascular tone and provide chronotropic stimulation to the heart.[8] Vasopressor treatment should not be taken lightly, as recent research has found an increased risk of complications associated with SCI and vasopressor administration, particularly dopamine and phenylephrine.[9] The evidence supports improved neurologic outcomes when mean arterial pressure (MAP) values greater than 85 mm Hg can be maintained in the first week following SCI.[7,10]

Concurrent with efforts to stabilize acute SCI patients, they should be transferred to specialized centers that can provide advanced trauma and spine care whenever possible. This is a level II recommendation in the 2013 Acute SCI Guidelines (**Table 5.1**).[5] It is increasingly recognized that medical outcomes are best when treatment occurs at specialized, high-volume centers.

Table 5.1 Abbreviated Guidelines for the Management of Acute Cervical Spine and Spinal Cord Injuries: 2013 update

Topic	Recommendation	Level of Evidence
Immobilization	Spinal immobilization of all trauma patients with a cervical spine or spinal cord injury or with a mechanism of injury having the potential to cause cervical spinal injury is recommended.	II
Immobilization	Triage of patients with potential spinal injury at the scene by trained and experienced EMS personnel to determine the need for immobilization during transport is recommended.	II
Immobilization	Immobilization of trauma patients who are awake, alert, and are not intoxicated, who are without neck pain or tenderness, who do not have an abnormal motor or sensory examination and who do not have any significant associated injury that might detract from their general evaluation is not recommended.	II
Immobilization	Spinal immobilization in patients with penetrating trauma is not recommended due to increased mortality from delayed resuscitation.	III
Transportation	Whenever possible, the transport of patients with acute cervical spine or spinal cord injuries to specialized acute spinal cord injury treatment centers is recommended.	III
Clinical assessment: neurological status	The ASIA international standards are recommended as the preferred neurologic examination tool.	II
Clinical assessment: functional status	The Spinal Cord Independence Measure (SCIM III) is recommended as the preferred functional outcome assessment tool for clinicians involved in the assessment, care, and follow-up of patients with spinal cord injuries.	I

(*continued*)

Table 5.1 (*continued*)

Topic	Recommendation	Level of Evidence
Clinical assessment: pain	The International Spinal Cord Injury Basic Pain Data Set (ISCIB-PDS) is recommended as the preferred means to assess pain including pain severity, physical functioning, and emotional functioning among SCI patients.	I
Radiographic assessment: asymptomatic patient	In the awake, asymptomatic patient who is without neck pain or tenderness, who has a normal neurologic examination, is without an injury detracting from an accurate evaluation, and who is able to complete a functional range of motion examination; radiographic evaluation of the cervical spine is not recommended.	I
Radiographic assessment: asymptomatic patient	Discontinuance of cervical immobilization for these patients is recommended without cervical spinal imaging.	I
Radiographic assessment: asymptomatic patient	In the awake patient with neck pain or tenderness and normal high-quality CT imaging or normal three-view cervical spine series (with supplemental CT if indicated), the following recommendations should be considered: (1) continue cervical immobilization until asymptomatic; (2) discontinue cervical immobilization following normal and adequate dynamic flexion/extension radiographs; (3) discontinue cervical immobilization following a normal MRI obtained within 48 hours of injury (limited and conflicting class II and class III medical evidence); or (4) discontinue cervical immobilization at the discretion of the treating physician.	III
Radiographic assessment: symptomatic patient	In the awake, symptomatic patient, high-quality CT imaging of the cervical spine is recommended.	I
Radiographic assessment: symptomatic patient	If high-quality CT imaging is available, routine three-view cervical spine radiographs are not recommended.	I
Radiographic assessment: symptomatic patient	If high-quality CT imaging is not available, a three-view cervical spine series (AP, lateral, and odontoid views) is recommended. This should be supplemented with CT (when it becomes available) if necessary to further define areas that are suspicious or not well visualized on the plain cervical X-rays.	I
Radiographic evaluation in obtunded (or unevaluable) patients	In the obtunded or unevaluable patient, high-quality CT imaging is recommended as the initial imaging modality of choice. If CT imaging is available, routine three-view cervical spine radiographs are not recommended.	I
Radiographic evaluation in obtunded (or unevaluable) patients	If high-quality CT imaging is not available, a three-view cervical spine series (AP, lateral, and odontoid views) is recommended. This should be supplemented with CT (when it becomes available) if necessary to further define areas that are suspicious or not well visualized on the plain cervical X-rays.	I
Closed reduction	Early closed reduction is recommended.	III
Cardiopulmonary management	Management of patients with acute SCI in a monitored setting is recommended.	III
Cardiopulmonary Management	Maintain mean arterial BP 85 to 90 mm Hg after SCI is recommended	III

Table 5.1 (*continued*)

Topic	Recommendation	Level of Evidence
Pharmacology management: corticosteroids*	Administration of methylprednisolone (MP) for the treatment of acute SCI is not recommended. Clinicians considering MP therapy should bear in mind that the drug is not FDA approved for this application. There is no class I or class II medical evidence supporting the clinical benefit of MP in the treatment of acute SCI. Scattered reports of class III evidence claim inconsistent effects likely related to random chance or selection bias. However, class I, II, and III evidence exists that high-dose steroids are associated with harmful side effects including death.	I
Pharmacology management: GM_1-ganglioside	Administration of GM_1-ganglioside (Sygen) for the treatment of acute SCI is not recommended.	I
Classification of subaxial injuries	SLIC and CSISS	I
Classification of subaxial cervical injuries	Harris and Allen	III
Subaxial cervical spinal injuries	The routine use of CT and MRI of trauma victims with ankylosing spondylitis is recommended, even after minor trauma.	III
Subaxial cervical spinal injuries	For patients with ankylosing spondylitis who require surgical stabilization, posterior long segment instrumentation and fusion, or a combined dorsal and anterior procedure, is recommended. Anterior stand-alone instrumentation and fusion procedures are associated with a failure rate of up to 50% in these patients.	III
Central cord syndrome	Aggressive multimodality management of patients with ATCCS is recommended.	III
Pediatric injuries: diagnostic	CT imaging to determine the condyle–C1 interval for pediatric patients with potential AOD is recommended.	I
Pediatric injuries: diagnostic	Cervical spine imaging is not recommended in children who are older than 3 years of age and who have experienced trauma and who (1) are alert, (2) have no neurologic deficit, (3) have no midline cervical tenderness, (4) have no painful distracting injury, (5) do not have unexplained hypotension, (6) and are not intoxicated. Cervical spine imaging is not recommended in children who are younger than 3 years of age and who have experienced trauma and who: (1) have a GCS > 13, (2) have no neurologic deficit, (3) have no midline cervical tenderness, (4) have no painful distracting injury, (5) are not intoxicated, (6) do not have unexplained hypotension, (7) were not in a motor vehicle collision (MVC), (8) suffered a fall from a height greater than 10 feet, (9) or suffered a nonaccidental trauma (NAT) as a known or suspected mechanism of injury.	II

(*continued*)

Table 5.1 (*continued*)

Topic	Recommendation	Level of Evidence
Pediatric injuries: diagnostic	Cervical spine radiographs or high-resolution CT is recommended for children who have experienced trauma and who do not meet either set of criteria above.	II
Pediatric injuries: diagnostic	Three-position CT with C1-C2 motion analysis to confirm and classify the diagnosis is recommended for children suspected of having atlanto-axial rotatory fixation (AARF).	II
Pediatric injuries: diagnostic	AP and lateral cervical spine radiography or high-resolution CT is recommended to assess the cervical spine in children younger than 9 years of age.	III
Pediatric injuries: diagnostic	AP, lateral, and open-mouth cervical spine radiography or high-resolution CT is recommended to assess the cervical spine in children 9 years of age and older.	III
Pediatric injuries: diagnostic	High-resolution CT scan with attention to the suspected level of neurologic injury is recommended to exclude occult fractures or to evaluate regions not adequately visualized on plain radiographs.	III
Pediatric injuries: diagnostic	Flexion and extension cervical radiographs or fluoroscopy are recommended to exclude gross ligamentous instability when there remains a suspicion of cervical spinal instability following static radiographs or CT scan.	III
Pediatric injuries: diagnostic	MRI of the cervical spine is recommended to exclude spinal cord or nerve root compression, evaluate ligamentous integrity, or provide information regarding neurologic prognosis.	III
Pediatric injuries: treatment	Reduction with manipulation or halter traction is recommended for patients with acute AARF (less than 4 weeks' duration) that does not reduce spontaneously. Reduction with halter or tong/halo traction is recommended for patients with chronic AARF (greater than 4 weeks' duration).	III
Pediatric injuries: treatment	Internal fixation and fusion are recommended in patients with recurrent and/or irreducible AARF.	III
Pediatric injuries: treatment	Operative therapy is recommended for cervical spine injuries that fail nonoperative management.	III
SCIWORA: diagnosis	MRI of the region of suspected neurologic injury is recommended in a patient with SCIWORA.	III
SCIWORA: diagnosis	Radiographic screening of the entire spinal column is recommended.	III
SCIWORA: diagnosis	Assessment of spinal stability in a SCIWORA patient is recommended, using flexion-extension radiographs in the acute setting and at late follow-up, even in the presence of a MRI negative for extraneural injury.	III
SCIWORA: treatment	External immobilization of the spinal segment of injury is recommended for up to 12 weeks.	III
SCIWORA: treatment	Early discontinuation of external immobilization is recommended for patients who become asymptomatic and in whom spinal stability is confirmed with flexion and extension radiographs.	III
SCIWORA: treatment	Avoidance of high-risk activities for up to 6 months following SCIWORA is recommended.	III
Vertebral artery injury: diagnostic	CTA is recommended as a screening tool in selected patients after blunt cervical trauma who meet the modified Denver Screening Criteria for suspected VAI.	I

Table 5.1 (*continued*)

Topic	Recommendation	Level of Evidence
Vertebral artery injury: diagnostic	Conventional catheter angiography is recommended for the diagnosis of VAI in selected patients after blunt cervical trauma, particularly if concurrent endovascular therapy is a potential consideration, and can be undertaken in circumstances in which CTA is not available.	III
Vertebral artery injury: diagnostic	MRI is recommended for the diagnosis of VAI after blunt cervical trauma in patients with a complete spinal cord injury or vertebral subluxation injuries.	III
Vertebral artery injury: treatment	It is recommended that the choice of therapy for patients with VAI, anticoagulation therapy vs antiplatelet therapy vs no treatment, be individualized based on the patient's vertebral artery injury, associated injuries, and risk of bleeding.	III
Vertebral artery injury: treatment	The role of endovascular therapy in VAI has yet to be defined; therefore, no recommendation regarding its use in the treatment of VAI can be offered.	III
Vertebral artery injury: treatment	Observation in patients with VAI and no evidence of posterior circulation ischemia is recommended.	III
Venous thromboembolism: prophylaxis	Early administration of VTE prophylaxis (within 72 hours) is recommended.	II
Venous thromboembolism: prophylaxis	Vena cava filters are not recommended as a routine prophylactic measure, but are recommended for select patients who fail anticoagulation or who are not candidates for anticoagulation or mechanical devices.	III
Nutritional support	Indirect calorimetry as the best means to determine the caloric needs of spinal cord injury patients is recommended.	II
Nutritional support	Nutritional support of SCI patients is recommended as soon as feasible. It appears that early enteral nutrition (initiated within 72 hours) is safe, but has not been shown to affect neurologic outcome, the length of stay, or the incidence of complications in patients with acute SCI.	III

Abbreviations: AOD, atlanto-occipital dissociation; AP, anteroposterior; ASIA, American Spinal Injury Association; ATCCS, acute traumatic central cord syndrome; CSISS, Cervical Spine Injury Severity Score; CT, computed tomography; CTA, computed tomographic angiography; EMS, emergency medical services; FDA, Food and Drug Administration; GCS, Glasgow Coma Scale; MPSS, methylprednisolone sodium succinate; MRI, magnetic resonance imaging; SCI, spinal cord injury; SCIWORA, spinal cord injury without radiographic abnormality; SLIC, Subaxial Cervical Spine Injury Classification; VAI, vertebral artery injury; VTE, venous thromboembolism.
* This guideline is controversial. New AOSpine guidelines recommend MPSS infusion for 24 hours as a treatment option if administered within 8 hours of injury.

Physical Examination and Clinical Assessment

Once the patient is stabilized and fully resuscitated, a detailed neurologic exam is performed. The American Spinal Injury Association (ASIA) classification, also known as the International Standard for Neurological Classification of Spinal Cord Injury (abbreviated as ISNCSCI), is the preferred tool for neurologic examination following an acute SCI (level II).[5] The classification categorizes patients into five grades (A to E) based on sensory and motor function and on whether the injury is complete or incomplete (**Table 5.2**).[11-14] Sacral sparing is critical to identify in these assessments, as it connotes an incomplete injury and portends a better prognosis.

Table 5.2 The 2011 Revised International Standard for Neurological Classification of Spinal Cord Injury ASIA Impairment Scale (AIS)

A = Complete	No sensory or motor function is preserved in the sacral segments S4-S5.
B = Sensory incomplete	Sensory but not motor function is preserved below the neurologic level and includes the sacral segments S4-S5, AND no motor function is preserved more than three levels below the motor level on either side of the body.
C = Motor incomplete	Motor function is preserved below the neurologic level, and more than half of key muscle functions below the single neurologic level of injury have a muscle grade less than 3 (grades 0–2).
D = Motor incomplete	Motor function is preserved below the neurologic level, and at least half (half or more) of key muscle functions below the neurologic level of injury have a muscle grade > 3.
E = Normal	If sensation and motor function as tested with the ISNCSCI are graded as normal in all segments, and the patient had prior deficits, then the AIS grade is E. Someone without a SCI does not receive an AIS grade.

Abbreviations: AIS, American Spinal Injury Association Impairment Scale; ISNCSCI, International Standards for Neurological Classification of Spinal Cord Injury; SCI, spinal cord injury.

▨ Imaging

In patients with traumatic neurologic deficits, imaging is required to define the anatomy of the injury. According to SCI guidelines, only patients with a possible diagnosis of SCI or those with altered mental status who are unable to comply with the neurologic exam require imaging (level I).[5] Initial imaging in any patient with an acute SCI should be a high-quality computed tomography (CT) scan (level I). If a CT scan is unavailable, X-rays are recommended and a CT scan should be performed when it becomes available (level I). A patient with cervical pain or tenderness despite normal imaging should have cervical immobilization continued until the patient is symptom free. Dynamic flexion/extension radiographs may then be used to exclude instability indicative of ligamentous injury. Magnetic resonance imaging (MRI) within 48 hours of injury may also provide reassurance that cervical immobilization can be discontinued (level III). Although CT scan is the preferred initial imaging modality, MRI is the most useful modality for identifying and characterizing spinal cord lesions. The utility of MRI for outcome prediction in patients with SCI is being increasingly recognized.[15]

▨ Spinal Cord Decompression

The SCI guidelines recommend early closed reduction of cervical fractures if possible (level III).[5] There are several contraindications to cervical traction, such as extension-distraction injury (especially in the context of ankylosing spondylitis), local infection, comminuted skull fracture, a hemodynamically unstable patient, atlanto-occipital dislocations, and depressed level of consciousness. Reviews have reported that 80% of patients with acute SCI dislocation were effectively reduced with closed decompression.[5] However, it has been reported that ~ 1% of patients with closed reduction suffer from permanent neurologic deficit, and 2 to 4% experience transient neurologic deficit.

There has been much controversy about the timing of decompression in acute SCI patients. Some studies have reported poor outcomes in acutely injured patients, and others have reported no neurologic advantage in early decompression (defined as less than 72 hour).[16] Researchers have also reported improved neurologic outcomes from early decompression of acute SCI when a more stringent definition of early is employed (8 to 24 hours).[5,16] The Surgical Timing in Acute Spinal Cord Injury Study

(STASCIS) is an important prospective observational study that provides the best evidence regarding the neurologic benefit inherent in early spinal cord decompression. Of the 313 patients who underwent decompression, 182 had surgery within 24 hours after the injury, and 20% of these patients improved by two or more ASIA Impairment Scale (AIS) grades at 6-month follow-up, which was statically greater than the 9% of patients who improved by two or more grades in the group undergoing decompression longer than 24 hours after the injury.[16] The STASCIS study found no significant difference in mortality or complications in either group, demonstrating the safety of early surgery. Of interest, a greater percentage of patients diagnosed with AIS grade A injuries improved in the early decompression groups than in the greater than 24 hours group (43% vs 37%, respectively), providing compelling reason to avoid skepticism regarding the value of early treatment in these patients. It is also noteworthy that a recent study found that patients with traumatic central cord syndrome may also benefit from early decompression (less than 24 hours after injury).[17] This is important given that many surgeons have historically preferred delayed decompression in these patients.

Neurocritical Care Management

Pharmacological Management

The SCI guidelines have made several changes to the pharmacological management of acute SCI patients. The 2002 SCI guidelines included the use of methylprednisolone sodium succinate (MPSS) as a treatment option.[5] Despite little change in the relevant evidence, the 2013 updated SCI guidelines recommend against the use of MPSS (level I recommendation).[5] This has proven to be a very controversial change.

Glucocorticoids have demonstrated neuroprotective properties following acute SCI as they decrease inflammation, protect cell membranes, and increase spinal cord blood flow.[2] MPSS was studied in the three large, high-quality National Acute Spinal Cord Injury Study (NASCIS) trials.[2,5] The NASCIS I trial studied two groups: one group of SCI patients received a 100-mg bolus of methylprednisolone followed by 10 days of treatment, and the other group received a 1,000-mg bolus followed by 10 days of treatment; no comparison was made to a placebo group.[2] The results from trial I showed no significant difference between the two groups in neurologic function at 42 days and 180 days post-SCI; however, animal studies conducted subsequent to the initiation of NASCIS I suggested that the employed doses were too small to be of benefit.[2]

The NASCIS II trial randomized acute SCI patients to three different groups: one group received an increased dose of methylprednisolone (30 mg/kg bolus followed by 5.4 mg/kg/h for the first day), a second group received naloxone, and a third group received a placebo.[2] Importantly, this was the only NASCIS study to include a placebo group. The study found significant neurologic improvement in patients receiving methylprednisolone within 8 hours of injury. In patients receiving methylprednisolone after 8 hours of injury, neurologic improvement was not apparent.

The NASCIS III trial was the only NASCIS trial to include a quality-of-life outcome measure. It had three experimental groups: the first group received the NASCIS II dosing of MPSS, the second group received high-dose MPSS, and the third group received a bolus of methylprednisolone followed by tirilazad mesylate (a 21-aminosteroid that functions as an antioxidant without glucocorticoid effects).[2] When treatment was initiated within 3 hours, no difference in neurologic outcomes was noted between groups; patients treated with high-dose MPSS demonstrated significantly improved neurologic function when treatment was begun between 3 and 8 hours after injury.[2] A substantial increase in complications, however, was seen with high-dose MPSS, prompting most practitioners to use NASCIS II dosing instead. Neurologic benefit was additionally noted in STASCIS patients who received MPSS, providing further evidence for its efficacy.[16] Many clinicians cite the small effect size and risk of complications as reasons for not prescribing

MPSS to those with acute SCI, although many still feel that its use is justified. Following a recent systematic review, the new guidelines generated by AOSpine will recognize the 24-hour infusion of MPSS as a treatment option, especially in patients with cervical SCI. However, the guidelines will recommend against 48-hour infusion of MPSS.

Of the numerous pharmacological agents studied in human SCI, the only other with suggested efficacy is GM_1-ganglioside. In the 2002 SCI guidelines, GM_1-ganglioside was recommended as a treatment option, although it was never made available for administration.[5] In the 2013 update, GM_1-ganglioside treatment is no longer recommended in acute SCI patients. GM_1-ganglioside in animal models has been shown to decrease neuronal cell death.

Complications

Respiratory Complications

Physicians must watch cervical SCI patients closely for respiratory insufficiency even when diaphragmatic function is intact. Hypoxia exacerbates neurologic damage following SCI and must be avoided. It has been found that 33% of cervical SCI patients require intubation within the first day and up to 90% require mechanical ventilation within the first 72 hours.[2] Patients must be observed for the use of accessory muscles of respiration including the intercostals, sternocleidomastoids, scalenes, and pectoralis major. These accessory muscles can also be denervated following a SCI. Paralysis of intercostal musculature is associated with a ~ 70% decrease in forced vital capacity and maximal inspiratory force because inspiration causes chest wall collapse until the onset of spasticity. Lung contusions, adult respiratory distress syndrome, pneumonia, and other pathologies can additionally compromise the respiratory function of SCI patients, so vigilance is critical. Initially when inhalation and exhalation are compromised in an SCI, the patient will compensate by increasing the rate of breathing (albeit with low tidal volumes). Patients who compensate initially may fatigue rapidly, becoming unable to maintain tachypnea sufficient to meet respiratory demands, thus becoming hypercarbic. When possible intubation should be performed in a nonemergent setting. It is thus useful to monitor vital capacity in cervical SCI patients; intubation should be considered in patients whose vital capacity is less than 1 L, particularly if there is evidence of fatigue. Intubation should also be considered in the context of respiratory distress, especially if the partial pressure of carbon dioxide in the arterial blood is high.

Typically, cervical SCI patients who require intubation experience improved respiratory function over the next 2 weeks.[2] Patients with lower cervical injury who initially need intubation frequently begin to gain rigidity in their intercostal muscles, enabling the chest wall to be supported. Published studies have correlated the number of days cervical SCI patients require mechanical ventilation with the level of injury and the degree to which the injury is incomplete. A complete injury requires mechanical ventilation for a longer duration than incomplete injuries. Mechanical ventilation was needed for an average of 65 days for high spinal cord injuries compared with 12 days for thoracic injuries. Tracheostomy should be strongly considered if mechanical ventilation is needed for longer than 14 days. Tracheostomy can assist ventilator weaning and lead to earlier discharge from the critical care unit.

Cardiovascular Complications

Spinal cord injury patients are vulnerable to a long list of possible cardiovascular abnormalities. Loss of sympathetic tone is a major concern in SCI above T6.[2] This lack of sympathetic outflow causes dominant parasympathetic tone leading to bradycardia and hypotension. Neurogenic shock thus results from a lack of tone in blood vessels, and pooling of blood in the periphery with a lack of return to the heart for distribution to tissues. As in all hypotensive patients, the first step in management is intravenous fluid administration. However, if after 1 to 2 L of IV fluids the blood pressure remains low, a vasopressor agent must be given, as these patients are susceptible to fluid overload.

Current SCI guidelines recommend maintaining MAP values above 85 to 90 mm Hg for

7 days following an acute SCI (level III).[5] To achieve this goal, patients almost universally require administration of pressors and management in a critical care unit. Although these recommendations are widely practiced, most of the research is from uncontrolled studies, and the 85 to 90 mm Hg threshold appears to have been selected arbitrarily.[2] A recent study by Hawryluk and colleagues[10] validated this recommendation with a data set of high-frequency physiological data. A strong inverse correlation was found between the amount of time MAP is below 85 mm Hg and neurologic improvement. The effect persisted for 5 to 7 days and decreased over time.

Another manifestation of the loss of sympathetic tone can be cardiac dysrhythmia.[2] In some studies severe cardiac dysrhythmias including arrest are seen in as many as 15% of cervical SCI patients.[2] The most common time for these dysthymias to occur is ~ 72 hours from the time of injury, but can be seen for up to 14 days. The bradycardia that typifies cervical SCI can be treated with a variety of medications including atropine and inotropes. When refractory to medications, a pacemaker may be needed. In a recent series, 17% of cervical SCI patients received a cardiac pacemaker.

Autonomic dysreflexia can also occur following SCI.[2] Typically, bladder or bowel distention causes a marked increase in sympathetic tone, which in turn causes hypertension and tachycardia. Autonomic dysreflexia may occur in up to 90% of quadriplegic patients. Although typically seen in the chronic stages of SCI, autonomic dysreflexia may occur in up to 3% of patients in the acute setting. Autonomic dysreflexia can have severe consequences, such as intracranial hemorrhage and even death. Treatment of this sympathetic overflow primarily involves removing the offending stimulus either by urinary catheter insertion for bladder distention or by enema for bowel distention. Symptomatic treatment may be needed, including rapidly acting antihypertensives.

Other Complications

Acute traumatic SCI patients are at risk for many complications due to their unique defi-

cits and because of their other injuries. Physicians should always consider the possibility of occult injuries that may go unnoticed due to sensory deficits. Intra-abdominal pathology such as hemorrhage, ruptured viscus, and sepsis are classically overlooked in these patients. A high index of suspicion is thus required.

Also, SCI patients are at very high risk for venous thrombosis secondary to tissue injury and venous stasis due to paralysis. This risk is even greater in the presence of additional injuries such as long bone fractures. The current literature reports an 81% risk of thromboembolism in SCI patients.[2] Most deep venous thromboses (DVTs) occurs between 3 days and 2 weeks after injury. The most recent SCI guidelines recommend low molecular weight heparin, rotating beds, pneumatic compressions stockings, and electrical compression devices for prophylaxis.[2,18] Inferior vena cava filters are recommended for patients who cannot be safely treated with prophylaxis or who have an existing deep venous thrombus and cannot start therapeutic anticoagulation. In total, 3 months of prophylaxis are recommended in SCI patients, with regular screening of extremities for DVT using clinical and laboratory assessments.[2,18] All patients with SCI need careful observation for signs of pulmonary embolism (PE) including chest pain, tachycardia, and increased oxygen demand. Spiral CT is the diagnostic test of choice in most facilities and has a sensitivity of 94% and specificity of 96%.[2] Once a patient is diagnosed with a PE anticoagulation needs to be administered.[2] A typical regimen is low molecular weight heparin for 5 days and warfarin until an international normalized ratio (INR) of between 2 to 3 is achieved and stable. Warfarin treatment is recommended for 6 months following a PE.

Pressure ulcers are a common complication in SCI patients, and constant surveillance and preventative measures are needed.[19] Prevention is strongly preferred due to the challenges inherent in the treatment of pressure ulcers. Prevention begins with pressure relief including frequent turning, special mattresses, heel protectors, and removal of any source of pressure. Once a pressure ulcer is formed, immediate treatment is recommended, which may entail surgical debridement. Proper nutrition is vital to healing of ulcers, and a dietician should be consulted.

Psychosocial issues often develop early in SCI patients, including delirium and depression. Psychosocial factors impact the recovery of SCI patients and need to be treated aggressively. Referral to mental health professionals and social workers may be needed. Initial interventions should focus on the acute care environment and aspects of life after injury.[20]

Future Directions

Numerous promising preclinical and clinical studies aiming to improve outcome from acute SCI are ongoing. Hypothermia has long been explored for its putative neuroprotective effects.[2] Rigorous scientific methodology has been lacking in the studies conducted to date. A large multicenter study is currently being conducted to investigate the role of hypothermia in acute SCI (Clinicaltrials.gov identifier NCT01739010). Myelin components have been shown to inhibit neurite regeneration following injury. Antagonists of these inhibitors include VA-210 (formerly Cethrin) as well as Nogo antagonist ATI-355. Riluzole is a neuroprotective drug approved for use in amyo-

trophic lateral sclerosis that is currently being studied in a human SCI clinical trial. The anti-inflammatory antibiotic minocycline has also shown promise in a phase II human trial. A combination of magnesium and polyethylene glycol is also being studied in a phase II trial. A fibroblast growth factor analogue and granulocyte colony-stimulating factor are also under study. Cellular transplantation performed for human SCI has employed various cell types, and the studies have varying goals and varying levels of scientific rigor. Transplanted cell types have included activated autologous macrophages, Schwann cells, olfactory ensheathing cells, bone marrow stromal cells, and human embryonic stem cells (**Table 5.3**).[21] There is also interest in cerebrospinal fluid drainage and monitoring, and treating spinal cord perfusion pressure.

Conclusion

Acute SCI continues to be a devastating disease that leaves many patients with permanent disability. It is increasingly evident that the quality of the supportive care received by SCI patients has a significant impact on their neurologic recovery. Indeed, improved critical care has markedly improved the outcomes from SCI

Table 5.3 Experimental Translational Treatments Currently Being Investigated for SCI

Translational Treatment	Phase	Clinicaltrials.gov Registration Information
Transplantation of autologous olfactory ensheathing cells	I	Not registered
Activated autologous macrophage implantation	I	Not registered
Bone marrow stromal cell transplantation	I/II	Not registered
Systemic hypothermia	I/II	NCT01739010
Minocycline treatment	II	Not registered
Riluzole treatment (sodium channel blockade and antiglutamatergic)	I	Not registered
ATI-355 (Nogo blockade)	I	NCT00406016
VA-210 (Cethrin) Treatment (Rho inhibition)	I/II	NCT00500812
Cerebrospinal fluid drainage for 72 hours	I	NCT00135278
Magnesium/polyethylene glycol combination	II	Not registered
Fibroblast growth factor analogue	I/II	NCT02490501
Granulocyte colony-stimulating factor	?	Not registered

in recent decades. Best care continues to evolve, and several promising therapeutics and therapeutic strategies hold promise for benefiting acute SCI patients in the near future. There is good reason for both patients and physicians to be optimistic.

literature has reported improved neurologic outcomes in patients undergoing early spinal cord decompression. This recognition has been an important advance. Additional advances are anticipated from research targeting secondary injury mediators or regenerative pathways; this research is currently in clinical trials.

Chapter Summary

Acute traumatic spinal cord injuries are life threatening and often cause permanent, severe neurologic deficits. The acute nonoperative management of traumatic spinal cord injuries is aimed at minimizing further damage and optimizing nutrient delivery to injured tissue. The management of such injuries begins on arrival of emergency medical services, with a focus on the Advanced Trauma Life Support protocol and transfer of patients to appropriate facilities with appropriate immobilization. In the trauma bay, resuscitation is performed and the primary survey is initiated in the following order of injury assessment: airway, breathing, circulation, disability, and exposure. Imaging must be performed on all possibly spinal cord injured patients. Many acute traumatic SCI patients require intubation and mechanical ventilation. Maintaining a MAP greater than 85 mm Hg for the first week improves neurologic recovery. Other complications such as DVT and PE are inherently common in acute traumatic SCI patients, but the risk of such complications can be reduced. Due to sensory loss, an SCI patient may have other occult injuries, and a high level of suspicion is essential. The recent

Pearls

- Any patient with the possibility of a SCI needs proper immobilization, and transfer to specialized facility is recommended.
- Initial management of acute traumatic SCI patients follows ATLS protocols, as in all trauma patients.
- Any patient with the possibility of a SCI requires CT imaging, and MRI should also be considered.
- Early decompression of an acute SCI has been associated with improved neurologic outcome.
- Intubation and mechanical ventilation is often required in cervical SCI patients; patients who initially compensate can deteriorate precipitously.
- Mean arterial pressure maintenance at greater than 85 mm Hg for the first week following acute traumatic spinal cord is associated with improved neurologic outcome and is recommended.

Pitfalls

- Complications are common in acute traumatic SCI patients, and clinicians must be alert for respiratory failure, hypotension, hypoxia, deep vein thrombosis, pulmonary embolism, pneumonia, decubitus ulcers, bowel and bladder dysfunction, and other occult injuries.
- Optimal management of acute traumatic SCI patients requires a specialized treatment facility with experience in treating such patients.

References
Five Must-Read References

1. Ma VY, Chan L, Carruthers KJ. Incidence, prevalence, costs, and impact on disability of common conditions requiring rehabilitation in the United States: stroke, spinal cord injury, traumatic brain injury, multiple sclerosis, osteoarthritis, rheumatoid arthritis, limb loss, and back pain. Arch Phys Med Rehabil 2014;95:986–995
2. Evans LT, Lollis SS, Ball PA. Management of acute spinal cord injury in the neurocritical care unit. Neurosurg Clin N Am 2013;24:339–347
3. Kwon BK, Tetzlaff W, Grauer JN, Beiner J, Vaccaro AR. Pathophysiology and pharmacologic treatment of acute spinal cord injury. Spine J 2004;4:451–464
4. American College of Surgeons. ATLS Advanced Trauma Life Support Program for Doctors, 7th ed. Chicago: American College of Surgeons; 2004
5. Resnick DK. Updated guidelines for the management of acute cervical spine and spinal cord injury. Neurosurgery 2013;72(2, Suppl 2):1

6. Binazzi B, Bianchi R, Romagnoli I, et al. Chest wall kinematics and Hoover's sign. Respir Physiol Neurobiol 2008;160:325–333
7. Ropper AE, Neal MT, Theodore N. Acute management of traumatic cervical spinal cord injury. Pract Neurol 2015;15:266–272
8. Ball PA. Critical care of spinal cord injury. Spine 2001;26(24, Suppl):S27–S30
9. Inoue T, Manley GT, Patel N, Whetstone WD. Medical and surgical management after spinal cord injury: vasopressor usage, early surgery, and complications. J Neurotrauma 2014;31:284–291
10. Hawryluk G, Whetstone W, Saigal R, et al. Mean arterial blood pressure correlates with neurological recovery after human spinal cord injury: analysis of high frequency physiologic data. J Neurotrauma 2015; 32:1958–1967
11. Kirshblum SC, Burns SP, Biering-Sorensen F, et al. International standards for neurological classification of spinal cord injury (revised 2011). J Spinal Cord Med 2011;34:535–546
12. American Spinal Injury Association. International Standards for Neurological Classification of Spinal Cord Injury, revised 2000. Atlanta: ASIA; 2008
13. Frankel HL, Hancock DO, Hyslop G, et al. The value of postural reduction in the initial management of closed injuries of the spine with paraplegia and tetraplegia. I. Paraplegia 1969;7:179–192
14. Tator CH, Rowed DW, Schwartz ML, eds. Sunnybrook Cord Injury Scales for Assessing Neurological Injury and Neurological Recovery in Early Management of Acute Spinal Cord Injury. New York: Raven Press; 1982:7
15. Bozzo A, Marcoux J, Radhakrishna M, Pelletier J, Goulet B. The role of magnetic resonance imaging in the management of acute spinal cord injury. J Neurotrauma 2011;28:1401–1411
16. Fehlings MG, Vaccaro A, Wilson JR, et al. Early versus delayed decompression for traumatic cervical spinal cord injury: results of the Surgical Timing in Acute Spinal Cord Injury Study (STASCIS). PLoS ONE 2012;7:e32037
17. Anderson KK, Tetreault L, Shamji MF, et al. Optimal timing of surgical decompression for acute traumatic central cord syndrome: a systematic review of the literature. Neurosurgery 2015;77(Suppl 4):S15–S32
18. Hadley MN, Walters BC, Grabb PA, et al. Guidelines for the management of acute cervical spine and spinal cord injuries. Clin Neurosurg 2002;49:407–498
19. Kruger EA, Pires M, Ngann Y, Sterling M, Rubayi S. Comprehensive management of pressure ulcers in spinal cord injury: current concepts and future trends. J Spinal Cord Med 2013;36:572–585
20. Consortium for Spinal Cord Medicine. Early acute management in adults with spinal cord injury: a clinical practice guideline for health-care professionals. J Spinal Cord Med 2008;31:403–479
21. Youmans J. Current status and future direction of management of spinal cord injury. In: Winn HR, ed. Youmans Neurological Surgery, 6th ed. Philadelphia: Saunders; 2011

6

Role and Timing of Surgery for Traumatic Spinal Cord Injury: What Do We Know and What Should We Do?

Christopher D. Witiw and Michael G. Fehlings

■ Introduction

Acute traumatic spinal cord injury (SCI) is an all too common occurrence with potentially devastating personal loss and societal costs resulting. The traumatic insult to the spinal column disrupts the normal osteoligamentous anatomy, leading to biomechanical instability and often sustained compressive forces on the spinal cord. Surgical intervention is undertaken to eliminate the compressive forces, restore normal alignment and reestablish stability of the spinal column, thereby mitigating the potential for ongoing dynamic injury to the spinal cord and maximizing the potential for neurologic recovery.

Thanks to exceptional research efforts in the basic science and clinical realms, a substantial body of evidence has been amassed regarding the role of surgical intervention in the acute setting. Despite this evidence, however, controversy still remains, most notably surrounding the timing of intervention. Recent high-quality clinical evidence has addressed many of the controversies but others still persist.

This chapter reviews the current evidence for surgical intervention after acute traumatic SCI and discusses the impact this evidence has on clinical decision making. The underlying pathophysiological processes of the injury frame the discussion of the role and timing of surgical decompression and stabilization. The current state of the literature on cervical, thoracic, and thoracolumbar SCI is reviewed, and particular attention is paid to three unique clinical scenarios that require special consideration: traumatic central cord syndrome, cervical facet dislocation, and SCI in the polytrauma patient.

■ Pathophysiology of Spinal Cord Injury

An understanding of the role of surgical intervention in acute SCI, and in particular the timing of the intervention, hinges upon an appreciation of the underlying pathophysiological processes. This section focuses on the mechanisms of the initial traumatic primary injury and the subsequent cascade of cellular destruction that constitutes the secondary phase of SCI. The subsequent discussion of the role and timing of surgery as a means to mitigate injury and improve neurologic recovery is based on these important cellular biological concepts.

Primary Injury

The primary injury phase of acute SCI occurs at the time of traumatic insult to the spinal cord. Mechanical forces lead to disruption of cell membranes, neuronal axons, and blood vessels.[1] Most commonly, contusive and compressive forces result from the loss of structural integrity of the spinal column, whereas other mechanisms of injury include shear and stretch forces from rapid acceleration-deceleration.[2]

Secondary Injury

Experimental evidence suggests that the final neurologic deficit results from a combination of the primary injury and a time-dependent cascade of pathophysiological processes following immediately after the initial impact, which constitute the secondary injury phase.[3] The early stages of the secondary injury phase are temporally classified into immediate (the first 2 hours after the injury), early acute (after the first 2 hours and up to 48 hours after the injury), and subacute (from day 3 up to 2 weeks).[1] These processes include disruption of the microvasculature and the resultant petechial white matter hemorrhage, cell death from membrane disruption, glutamate excitotoxicity, and ionic dysregulation from Na^+ and Ca^{2+} influx. Ischemia from local vasospasm and thrombosis, which may be compounded by systemic autonomic dysregulation, lead to cellular hypoxia and further cell death.[4]

▪ Role and Timing of Surgery

Persistent compression and dynamic effects from spinal column instability are thought to be key contributors to secondary injury. Intervening during the immediate or early acute phases holds promise to improve neurologic outcomes by removing the compressive forces and mitigating the potential for further injury by stabilizing the spinal column (**Fig. 6.1**). This notion has spurred considerable preclinical research efforts to elucidate the association between neurologic outcomes and the role and timing of decompression. These efforts have now been translated into the clinical realm, and high-quality evidence is available to guide clinical decision making. This section briefly reviews the preclinical evidence and discusses the evidence available from clinical studies.

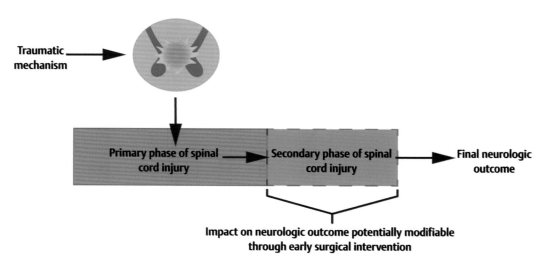

Fig. 6.1 A conceptual model of the impact of primary and secondary phases of spinal cord injury on neurologic recovery. Early surgical intervention holds promise to mitigate the deleterious effects of the secondary injury phase by eliminating the compressive forces on the spinal cord and providing stabilization to prevent ongoing dynamic traumatic forces.

There is more, and higher quality, clinical evidence relating to cervical SCI than is available for thoracic and thoracolumbar SCI, and so these areas will be treated separately.

Preclinical Evidence

Findings from numerous preclinical investigations support a time-dependent effect of spinal cord compression. Dimar et al[5] used a rat model with timed compression up to 72 hours and found better neurologic outcomes with shorter compression times. Carlson and colleagues,[6] using a dog model, compared compression times of 30 minutes and 3 hours, and found that subjects with 3 hours of compression had both worse neurologic outcome and greater lesion volumes. A recent meta-analysis of the preclinical literature suggests that outcome following acute SCI appears to be closely associated with the compressive pressure and duration, and that early decompression is an effective therapeutic strategy.[7] Overall the body of preclinical evidence supports a biological rationale for early spinal cord decompression through mitigation of the pathophysiological secondary injury processes.[8]

Clinical Evidence

Cervical Spine

Despite the preclinical support for early decompression, the association between timing of decompression and improved neurologic outcomes was not found to hold in early clinical studies of cervical SCI.[9,10] These studies had notable methodological limitations; for example, they used a time frame of 72 hours postinjury to distinguish early from late surgery, whereas evidence compiled from the literature as well as consensus expert opinion suggests that 24 hours postinjury is a more appropriate definition of early surgery.[8,11]

To provide high-quality evidence pertaining to the role of surgery within this 24-hour cutoff, the Surgical Timing in Acute Spinal Cord Injury Study (STASCIS) was initiated.[12] This international, multicenter, prospective cohort study included 313 patients with acute cervical SCI from six centers. Groups were compared through multivariate analysis, controlling for baseline differences. The analysis found that the odds of at least a two-grade improvement in the American Spinal Injury Association (ASIA) Impairment Scale (AIS) was 2.8 times higher at 6-month follow-up in the group that had early surgical decompression (**Fig. 6.2**). Moreover, the analysis of the outcomes data suggests that there may be a synergistic neuroprotective effect from the administration of methylprednisolone sodium succinate and early surgical decompression.[12] One of the primary criticisms of this trial is that there was a larger proportion of patients with AIS grade A or B injuries in the early surgery group, which favors the potential for an improvement of two or more grades.[13] Despite this limitation, the data provided by STASCIS represent the largest prospective investigation to date on the role of timing for surgical decompression in cervical SCI.

Based on the encouraging results of this trial, we believe that all patients with cervical SCI should have expedited imaging upon arrival at the hospital. Decompression should be undertaken in a manner appropriate for the nature of the patient's injury immediately following imaging, as long as the patient is stable from a hemodynamic and respiratory perspective.

Thoracic and Thoracolumbar Spine

The timing of surgical intervention for acute SCI secondary to injury of the thoracic or thoracolumbar spinal column has not received the same attention as that for the cervical spine. The evidence that is available suggests that early (< 72 hours) surgical stabilization of thoracic fractures may reduce the number of days on respiratory support, the length of stay in the critical care unit, the length of the overall hospital stay, and the mortality rate, when compared with late stabilization.[14,15] A small, single-center study of patients undergoing thoracolumbar stabilization with neurologic deficits for an acute thoracolumbar spinal injury found that patients having surgical decompression within 8 hours had significantly better postoperative AIS motor scores compared with those with late decompression.[16]

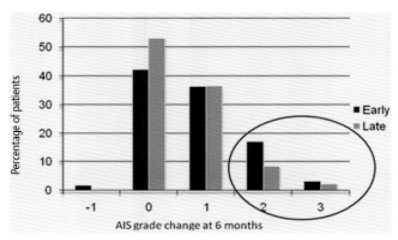

Fig. 6.2 Comparison of American Spinal Injury Association (ASIA) Impairment Scale (AIS) grade improvement at 6-month follow-up between patients undergoing early surgical decompression (< 24 hours) and those undergoing late decompression. It was found that 19.8% of patients in the early surgical group showed an improvement of two or more grades compared with only 8.8% in the late decompression group (odds ratio [OR], 2.57; 95% confidence interval, 1.11–5.97). (Reproduced from Fehlings MG, Vaccaro A, Wilson JR, et al. Early versus delayed decompression for traumatic cervical spinal cord injury: results of the Surgical Timing in Acute Spinal Cord Injury Study (STASCIS). PLoS ONE 2012; 7:e32037.)

Overall, the data available on the impact of early surgical intervention on this patient population suggest an improvement in several outcome measures. Although the strength and quality of evidence is not on a par with that for cervical SCI, we recommend a similar approach, favoring surgical intervention before 24 hours.

Focused Clinical Considerations

We support that overall tenet that patients with acute traumatic SCI should have surgical intervention as early as possible; however, three subgroups of patients present unique challenges that are addressed in this section.

Central Cord Syndrome

Surgical decision making for patients with central cord syndrome (CCS) is challenging because these patients often do not present evidence of overt spinal column instability, and spontaneous neurologic improvement may be observed. In cases of CCS associated with unstable injury to the spinal column or intervertebral disk herni-

ation, it is generally agreed that surgical intervention should be undertaken, but in cases where CCS results from the classic mechanism of hyperextension in the setting of cervical spondylosis without evidence of instability, many surgeons question if surgical intervention is warranted. A 2013 systematic review of the literature found four small, single-center, retrospective studies that compared surgical management with conservative management in patients with traumatic CCS.[17] Three of the studies demonstrated the superiority of surgery over conservative management in terms of neurologic recovery, but the study populations were quite heterogeneous and included unstable traumatic injuries as well as stable hyperextension-type injuries.

In those patients for whom surgical intervention is undertaken, controversy also exists regarding the timing of surgical intervention. The four studies cited above used varying timings to qualify as early surgery, ranging from less than 24 hours to less than 2 weeks.[17] Only one of the studies found a significant association between the timing of surgical intervention and neurologic outcome, and that study used the 2-week definition of early surgical intervention. Overall, there is a need for high-quality prospective studies to address the important relation between early surgery and neurologic outcomes. The Conservative or Early Surgical Management of Incomplete Cervical Cord Syndrome Without Spinal Instability (COSMIC) trial holds promise for providing higher quality evidence regarding the role of early surgical decompression (ClinicalTrials.gov identifier NCT01367405) for traumatic CCS. This multicenter randomized controlled trial, initiated in 2013, is designed to compare the clinical outcome of early (< 24 hours) surgery with that of conservative management.

Until higher quality evidence is available to guide clinical decision making, we believe that patients with traumatic CCS who have severe neurologic deficits (AIS grade C or worse) should have decompression within 24 hours if there is any magnetic resonance imaging (MRI) evidence of ongoing spinal cord compression or unstable osteoligamentous injury. The evidence for surgical intervention within 24 hours for patients with less severe neurologic injury is not as compelling. These patients should undergo decompressive surgery, but our time frame for intervention in such cases is within a week from the injury.

Cervical Facet Dislocation

Unilateral or bilateral cervical facet dislocations frequently present with injury to the spinal cord. Patients with facet dislocation have been found to have longer hospital stays and poorer recovery of motor function at 1 year following injury when compared with those with SCI without facet dislocation, even though decompression is generally performed sooner (25.1 hours versus 41.3 hours, respectively).[18] Despite this, ultra-early decompression potentially may hold promise for meaningful recovery. In an interesting case series, reported by Newton et al,[19] of rugby players with cervical facet dislocation, five of eight players with complete SCI who were reduced within 4 hours made a full neurologic recovery, whereas none of the 24 who were reduced after 4 hours achieved a similar recovery.

Fortunately, this injury pattern is generally amenable to decompression by reduction through closed means using Gardner-Wells tongs or a halo ring and incremental application of weight-based traction with serial monitoring by lateral radiographs and clinical examination (**Fig. 6.3**). In patients who are awake and cooperative, without distracting injuries, skull fractures, or evidence of atlanto-occipital dislocation, this treatment can typically be performed in an expedited manner. Once reduced, the spinal column should be stabilized with either halo vest application or continued traction of 20 lb until open surgical stabilization can be performed.

The need for MRI prior to closed reduction is still debated.[20] Concern exists that attempted closed reduction in the setting of traumatic intervertebral disk herniation could lead to progressive neurologic decline. Others believe that waiting for an MRI is a source of delay, and that transferring the patient to the MRI suite risks further injury. It is estimated that one third to one half of patients with cervical facet subluxation injuries demonstrate a disrupted or herniated intervertebral disk, but such a finding does not clearly influence neurologic outcome in closed reduction.[21]

We believe that MRI should be obtained prior to closed reduction in the setting of cervical facet dislocation with SCI, as long as it can be accessed in an expedited and safe manner. The patient should be monitored closely throughout the reduction procedure, and if there is any change in neurologic status, the procedure should be immediately halted, the spine immobilized, and emergent MRI performed, if not yet done, prior to taking the patient to the operating room for open reduction.

Polytrauma Patients with Spinal Cord Injury

Managing patients with SCI and other concurrent traumatic injuries presents considerable challenges. Often the neurologic exam is confounded by numerous factors, including

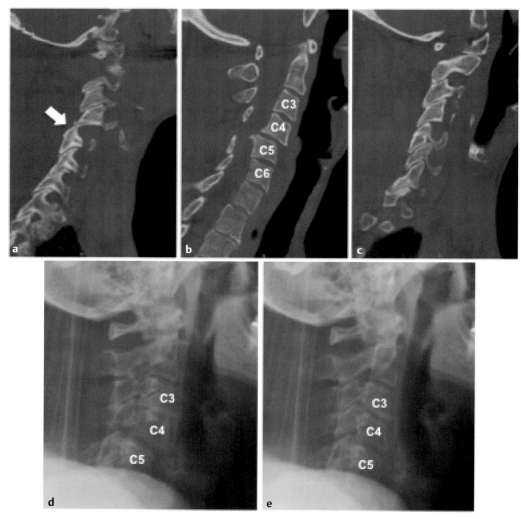

Fig. 6.3 A patient with a unilateral C4-C5 facet dislocation secondary to a high-speed motor vehicle collision. **(a)** Right parasagittal cuts from the initial computed tomography (CT) scan of the cervical spine at the time of presentation demonstrating C4-C5 facet dislocation *(arrow)*. **(b)** Midsagittal CT cuts demonstrating C4-C5 traumatic anterolisthesis. **(c)** Left parasagittal CT cuts. **(d)** Supine lateral cross-table radiographs of the cervical spine demonstrating C4-C5 misalignment prior to closed reduction. **(e)** Restoration of alignment following closed reduction with 25 lb of traction.

obtundation from intoxication or concurrent brain injury, sedation, extremity fractures, peripheral nerve injury, or a myriad of other circumstances. Furthermore, these patients may present in extremis from cardiorespiratory instability, necessitating immediate lifesaving intervention.

In the immediate period, a systematic approach to rapid assessment and institution of life-preserving therapy should be initiated in accordance with the Advanced Trauma Life Support Guidelines.[22] The heterogeneity of this patient population precludes establishing a single recommendation applicable to all patients regarding the role and timing of surgical intervention. Instead, clinical experience and acumen come to the forefront of decision making in these challenging scenarios. However there is some evidence available to help guide clinical decisions.

The STASCIS included patients with concurrent injuries, but the focus of the study was not on polytrauma patients. In addition, patients with life-threatening injuries that prevented early decompression of the spinal cord were excluded from the study.[12] Investigations that focused specifically on polytrauma patients generally used 72 hours as the dividing line between early and late surgery, and they used more general measures of outcome rather than neurologic recovery. Scaramuzzo et al[23] found that early fixation (< 72 hours) was associated with shorter length of critical care admission, shorter hospital stay, fewer days on mechanical ventilation, and less need for blood transfusion. In keeping with these findings, Chipman et al[24] reported a lower frequency of all complications in patients with an Injury Severity Score greater than 15 and receiving surgery within 72 hours of injury.

Although the evidence for the impact of early surgical intervention on neurologic recovery specifically in polytrauma patients is lacking, the available literature supports an improvement in overall metrics and decreased complications with early surgery. We suggest that surgical intervention should be undertaken in an expedited manner (< 24 hours) when there is evidence of neurologic deficit from SCI on clinical exam or compression on MRI. Factors that should add immediacy to increase the urgency of surgical decompression are cervical SCI, incomplete neurologic deficit, and evidence of progressive decline in neurologic function. However, a consensus that surgical intervention is safe must be reached among the multidisciplinary team tasked with managing the patient's current condition.

Chapter Summary

The mechanical forces associated with trauma to the spinal cord lead to primary injury through immediate disruption of cell membranes, neuronal axons, and blood vessels. This is followed by a time-dependent cascade of local pathobiological processes that comprise the secondary phase of SCI. Preclinical studies suggest that neurologic outcome is an aggregate of the primary injury and the progressive effects of secondary injury. There is a strong biological rationale for surgical intervention during the early acute secondary phase to remove compression and mitigate the dynamic traumatic effects of spinal column instability. This is in keeping with the principle that "time is spine."

Multicenter, prospective clinical studies in patients with cervical SCI support the findings of these preclinical studies. Surgical decompression within 24 hours of injury is associated with significant improvements in neurologic outcome. Although the evidence is not as strong for early decompression in patients with thoracic and thoracolumbar SCI, smaller clinical series have demonstrated a benefit on multiple measures of outcome. We believe, as a general principle, that patients with traumatic SCI should have surgical intervention as early as possible.

The subgroup of cervical SCI patients presenting with traumatic CCS are uniquely challenging because they often are without evidence of overt instability and may improve spontaneously. Until high-quality evidence to the contrary is available, we believe that these patients should have decompression within 24 hours if they present with severe neurologic injury (AIS grade C or worse). The evidence for decompression within the first 24 hours for patients with less severe neurologic injury is less compelling, and in these cases we generally do surgery within the first week from the time of injury. Two other subgroups of patients present unique challenges: cervical facet dislocation patients and SCI in polytrauma patients. Cervical facet dislocation should be managed rapidly with closed reduction, but there is controversy as to whether MRI should be obtained prior to reduction. We suggest obtaining imaging if it will not significantly delay treatment. The assessment of polytrauma patients necessitates a high degree of suspicion for SCI because the clinical exam may be confounded. Patients with polytrauma are challenging because concurrent injuries may preclude spinal surgery. If

SCI is identified, surgical intervention should be performed as early as possible, ideally within 24 hours, but only after ensuring safety through a consensus of the multidisciplinary trauma team.

Pearls

- Substantial preclinical evidence supports the biological rationale for early surgical decompression to mitigate the deleterious effects of the secondary injury phase of acute SCI.
- Prospective clinical studies in patients with cervical SCI suggest that surgical decompression performed within 24 hours results in improved neurologic outcomes. We support surgical intervention as soon as possible for these patients.
- There is some evidence that urgent decompression of the cervical spinal cord may synergistically enhance the impact of neuroprotective medications including methylprednisolone in cervical spinal cord injury.
- Although high-quality clinical evidence is not available to address the impact of early surgery for patients with thoracic or thoracolumbar SCI, early decompression is associated with improvements in multiple outcome measures, and we suggest that surgery be performed as soon as possible and at least within 24 hours.

- High-quality evidence is lacking for the role and timing of surgical intervention in patients with traumatic central cord syndrome. We suggest that surgery be performed within 24 hours for any patient with severe neurologic injury (AIS grade C or worse), whereas we generally operate within the first week of injury for patients with a less severe injury.

Pitfalls

- Magnetic resonance imaging should be obtained prior to performing a closed reduction in patients with cervical facet dislocations if it can be obtained in an expedited manner but not if it will significantly delay treatment.
- Patients undergoing closed reduction of cervical facet dislocations should be monitored closely, and the reduction should be halted with any change in neurologic status, and the patient then should be taken to the operating room for open reduction.
- The neurologic exam may be confounded by a myriad of factors in polytrauma patients but a high degree of suspicion for SCI will facilitate early recognition, and surgical intervention should be performed within 24 hours of injury as long as it is deemed safe by all members of the multidisciplinary trauma team.

References
Five Must-Read References

1. Rowland JW, Hawryluk GW, Kwon B, Fehlings MG. Current status of acute spinal cord injury pathophysiology and emerging therapies: promise on the horizon. Neurosurg Focus 2008;25:E2
2. Sekhon LH, Fehlings MG. Epidemiology, demographics, and pathophysiology of acute spinal cord injury. Spine 2001;26(24, Suppl):S2–S12
3. Carlson GD, Gorden C. Current developments in spinal cord injury research. Spine J 2002;2:116–128
4. Rossignol S, Schwab M, Schwartz M, Fehlings MG. Spinal cord injury: time to move? J Neurosci 2007;27:11782–11792
5. Dimar JR II, Glassman SD, Raque GH, Zhang YP, Shields CB. The influence of spinal canal narrowing and timing of decompression on neurologic recovery after spinal cord contusion in a rat model. Spine 1999;24:1623–1633
6. Carlson GD, Gorden CD, Oliff HS, Pillai JJ, LaManna JC. Sustained spinal cord compression: part I: time-dependent effect on long-term pathophysiology. J Bone Joint Surg Am 2003;85-A:86–94

7. Batchelor PE, Wills TE, Skeers P, et al. Meta-analysis of pre-clinical studies of early decompression in acute spinal cord injury: a battle of time and pressure. PLoS ONE 2013;8:e72659
8. Furlan JC, Noonan V, Cadotte DW, Fehlings MG. Timing of decompressive surgery of spinal cord after traumatic spinal cord injury: an evidence-based examination of pre-clinical and clinical studies. J Neurotrauma 2011;28:1371–1399
9. Vaccaro AR, Daugherty RJ, Sheehan TP, et al. Neurologic outcome of early versus late surgery for cervical spinal cord injury. Spine 1997;22:2609–2613
10. McKinley W, Meade MA, Kirshblum S, Barnard B. Outcomes of early surgical management versus late or no surgical intervention after acute spinal cord injury. Arch Phys Med Rehabil 2004;85:1818–1825
11. Fehlings MG, Rabin D, Sears W, Cadotte DW, Aarabi B. Current practice in the timing of surgical intervention in spinal cord injury. Spine 2010;35(21, Suppl):S166–S173

of MPSS, nimodipine, or both versus no pharmacological treatment, when administered within 8 hours of injury.[15] The trial enlisted 106 patients in a randomized fashion. Neurologic examinations at admission and 1 year later were performed using the American Spinal Injury Association (ASIA). Patients who were administered MPSS received it at a dose of 30 mg/kg over 1 hour followed by 5.4 mg/kg/h for 23 hours. At 1 year postinjury, there was no significant difference in ASIA scores between the treatment groups; 46% treated with MPSS experienced hyperglycemia compared with 3% of those who did not receive it, which was a significant difference. Overall, the lack of significant effect of MPSS administration on neurologic recovery as compared with no pharmacological treatment goes against the findings of the NASCIS II trial, which used the same dose of MPSS and protocol as this study. However, one could argue that the number of patients in this study was relatively small and potentially underpowered.

Another study by Matsumoto et al[16] aimed to perform a randomized controlled trial assessing the complications of high-dose therapy with MPSS compared with placebo in patients with acute SCI. Patients with cervical SCI were either administered MPSS according to the NASCIS II protocol or given placebo. There were 23 patients in both groups. Significant differences were observed in terms of pulmonary complications (eight cases in the MPSS group vs one case in the placebo group; $p = 0.009$) and gastrointestinal complications (four cases in the MPSS group vs 0 cases in the placebo group; $p = 0.036$) between the two groups. The authors concluded that patients with cervical SCI may experience pulmonary and gastrointestinal complications, but they do concede that the number of patients studied was small. Furthermore, there were a greater number of patients with less severe SCI in the placebo group compared with the treatment group, which could have also played a role in reducing complications observed in the placebo group. Overall, confirmatory trials performed after NASCIS II demonstrate conflicting results that may indicate decreased benefit for the use of methylprednisolone, but unfortunately, these studies suffer from various issues that make a robust recommendation against methylprednisolone difficult.

Cochrane Review

A Cochrane Review for the use of steroids in acute SCI was published in 2012.[17] Eight trials were found that address steroid therapy in acute SCI, and seven of them addressed MPSS. Overall, there was no effect found when comparing MPSS versus placebo or no treatment using the NASCIS II protocol. When only patients treated within 8 hours were included, high-dose MPSS treatment demonstrated greater motor function recovery at final outcome (6 months or 1 year, depending on the study) with a mean weighted difference of 4.06 (95% CI, 0.58–7.55) compared with placebo/no treatment (**Fig. 7.1**). With respect to the beneficial effect of extending MPSS therapy from 24 hours to 48 hours, the NASCIS III trial was the only study to address this issue in the Cochrane Review, so there were no other findings other than those demonstrated in the original trial. There was no difference in all-cause mortality between the MPSS and placebo/no treatment groups in the Cochrane Review. The pooled risk ratio of death from all causes at less than 180 days postinjury actually favored MPSS treatment at 0.54 (95% CI, 0.24–1.25). There were also no significant differences found in terms of wound infection and gastrointestinal hemorrhage between patients treated with MPSS and patients not treated. Overall, the conclusion of the review was that high-dose MPSS is the only pharmacological therapy with efficacy in a phase 3 randomized trial if started within 8 hours of injury, with additional benefit to extending the maintenance dose to 48 hours postinjury if it is started between 3 and 8 hours postinjury.

STASCIS

Wilson et al[18] assessed the complications associated with acute cervical SCI using the database for the Surgical Timing in Acute Spinal Cord Injury Study (STASCIS). STASCIS provided evidence that there may be neurologic benefit

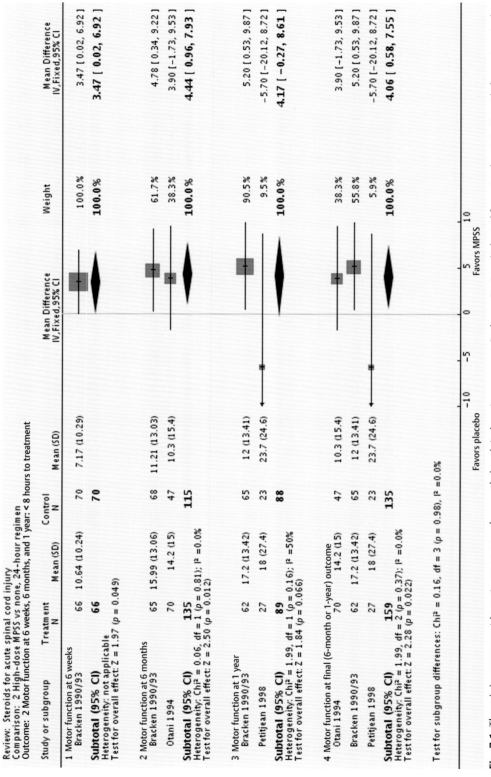

Fig. 7.1 There is improvement in motor recovery when methylprednisolone is given within 8 hours after spinal cord injury, as initially demonstrated in the National Acute Spinal Cord Injury Study (NASCIS) II trial and confirmed in a recent Cochrane Review. (Adapted from Bracken MB. Steroids for acute spinal cord injury. Cochrane Database Syst Rev 2012;1:CD001046.)

Table 7.1 Data from the Surgical Timing in Acute Spinal Cord Injury Study (STASCIS)

Predictor Variable	Odds Ratio	95% Confidence Interval	p Value
Patient age	1.02	1.00–1.03	0.047
Admission AIS grade			< 0.01
A	9.44	4.90–18.16	
B	4.76	2.22–10.18	
C	2.00	0.95–4.19	
D*	1.00		
Steroid administration	0.56	0.35–0.90	0.02
Comorbid illness			0.02
No	0.46	0.24–0.91	
Yes*	1.00		
High- vs low-energy injury mechanism	1.57	0.96–2.56	0.07

Abbreviation: AIS, American Spinal Injury Association Impairment Scale.
Source: From Wilson JR, Arnold PM, Singh A, Kalsi-Ryan S, Fehlings MG. Clinical prediction model for acute inpatient complications after traumatic cervical spinal cord injury: a subanalysis from the Surgical Timing in Acute Spinal Cord Injury Study. J Neurosurg Spine 2012;17(1, Suppl):46–51. Reprinted by permission.
Note: The data suggest that there may be potential synergy between early decompressive surgery and steroid administration after spinal cord injury. Results from multivariate logistic regression model predicting complication development. Predictors with a *p* value <.10 were retained.
*Reference category.

with early surgical decompression (within 24 hours) after SCI.[4] In the assessment of complications, 411 patients were analyzed for cardiopulmonary, surgical, thrombotic, infectious, and decubitus ulcer development. It was found that there were five predictors of complication development (*p* < 0.10), including the absence of steroid administration (odds ratio [OR], 0.56; 95% CI, 0.35–0.90; *p* = 0.02; **Table 7.1**). Given that many of the patients underwent early surgical decompression, it was postulated that there may be a synergy between surgery and steroid administration in reducing complications after SCI. The multivariate regression model developed in the original STASCIS report also demonstrated that surgical timing, complete versus incomplete status of SCI, and steroid administration predicted neurologic recovery at 6-month follow-up.[4] Although there may be certain caveats including the fact that STASCIS only looked at cervical SCI patients, for whom wound infection rates may be lower than in thoracic or lumbar surgical patients, in addition to the fact that the study's primary analysis was not focused on comparing patients treated with steroids versus not treated with

steroids, it does shed light on the possibility of synergy between surgery and steroid administration that is not addressed in the most recent guidelines.

Overall, the evidence regarding the use of methylprednisolone in SCI is mixed. However, there is some evidence in the form of randomized controlled trials and the recent Cochrane meta-analysis, which was not included in the recent guidelines, that demonstrate that methylprednisolone results in significant improvements in motor function when given within 8 hours postinjury for 24 hours postinjury, and that this effect is improved when given for 48 hours starting between 3 and 8 hours postinjury. The use of methylprednisolone has also not been shown to be definitively associated with greater mortality or complications.

Examination of the Current Guidelines

Two iterations of practice guidelines produced jointly by the AANS/CNS Spine Section for the management of SCI have provided contrasting recommendations for the use of methylprednisolone. In 2002, the guidelines suggested that methylprednisolone be used as an option in SCI but only with the knowledge that the evidence for harmful effects is more consistent than the suggestion of clinical benefit.[19] In 2013, the guidelines changed, making a level I recommendation against the administration of methylprednisolone in acute SCI.[20] However, looking at the evidence that has developed since 2002, we argue that it does not necessarily justify a change in recommendations.

Nine new studies on methylprednisolone were included in the 2013 guidelines that were published since the last iteration. These studies were a mixture of level II and level III evidence.[20] Three of the new studies demonstrated that patients treated with MPSS had better neurologic improvement. Lee et al[21] performed a retrospective review of 111 patients with SCI, and reported that subanalysis of patients with complete SCI who underwent surgery demonstrated that 11 of 16 patients treated with MPSS improved, whereas none of the seven patients who did not receive MPSS improved. Tsutsumi et al[22] demonstrated in their retrospective review of 70 cervical SCI patients treated over 5 years that there was recovery of 18 more ASIA scale motor points in patients who received MPSS compared with controls at 6 months ($p = 0.005$). Aito et al[23] demonstrated in a retrospective review of 65 patients over 24 years that the presence of neurologic improvement was more likely in patients treated with MPSS versus those not treated ($p = 0.005$). Similarly, three studies demonstrated more complications with MPSS. There was a significantly higher incidence of infection ($p = 0.028$) reported by Ito et al[24]; respiratory infection, total infection and early hyperglycemia reported by Suberviola et al[25]; and acute corticosteroid myopathy[26] in a prospective case-control cohort study of five SCI patients treated with MPSS and three patients not receiving MPSS, with no increased mortality reported with MPSS administration.

Again, the results regarding MPSS administration since 2002 have been mixed. Regardless, the presence of nonrandomized comparative studies, one can argue, does not provide enough

evidence for a level I recommendation against the use of steroids. Only the study by Leypold et al[27] was properly adjusted for baseline neurologic status, which has been shown to be a strong predictor of future neurologic and complication-related outcomes. In contrast, there has been evidence from the NASCIS trials and Cochrane Review, which arguably represent the highest levels of evidence, of the possible benefit of the use of MPSS in SCI.

The heterogeneity of SCI also remains an issue that has not been fully addressed in the recent guidelines. More specifically, it is unclear if different levels of SCI respond differently to MPSS therapy. A recent study by Evaniew et al[28] attempted to address this question. They looked at patients in the Rick Hansen Spinal Cord Injury Registry who received MPSS according to the NASCIS II protocol, using propensity score matching to account for, among other things, the neurologic level of injury. They found that MPSS did not result in improvement in motor score recovery in either the cervical or thoracic spine when anatomic level and severity of injury were included in the analysis. Ultimately, the study suffers from low numbers of patients, with only 46 patients analyzed who received MPSS, so robust conclusions in this regard are difficult to make. The heterogeneity of SCI still remains an issue that has not been fully addressed in the context of MPSS administration. Furthermore, this issue has not been clearly outlined in the recent guidelines against MPSS administration.

■ Chapter Summary

Based on the available data, we argue that MPSS should continue to be recommended as a treatment option, particularly for cervical SCI patients undergoing surgical decompression. Since 2002, the new evidence that has emerged involves nonrandomized comparative studies with inherent risks of bias, lack of control for baseline neurologic status, and demonstrated benefits of MPSS without increased mortality—all of which do not necessarily support a strict recommendation against the use of steroids in

Fig. 8.1 (*opposite*) Longitudinal and cross-sectional representation of the spinal cord at various stages following spinal cord injury. **(a)** Normal cord. **(b)** Immediate/acute injury. This phase is characterized by severing of axons at the epicenter and demyelination due to the primary injury. Gray matter hemorrhaging and small white matter hemorrhages are common. Necrosis of gray matter glia and sensory *(red)*, autonomic *(green)*, and motor neurons *(blue)* occurs, along with axonal swelling and accumulation of A-β protein (indicative of axonal transport failure). Microglia become activated due to necrotic by-products, and they secrete inflammatory cytokines and nitric oxide, further damaging tissue and recruiting systemic inflammatory cells. Necrosis of sympathetic preganglionic neurons *(green)* causes autonomic dysfunction. **(c)** Subacute injury. Hemorrhaging and edema continue, resulting in a spread of the hypoperfused/ischemic zone *(red area)*. This continues the necrosis and begins apoptotic cell death. Macrophages *(green)* infiltrate, contributing to the local damage. At the epicenter, acute necrosis of lower motor neuronal cell bodies results in degradation of the leftover axons *(blue dashed line)*. Severing of first-order sensory axons causes dieback toward the cell body (dorsal root ganglion, DRG). Severing of upper motor neuronal axons at the epicenter results in degradation of the distal end (*blue dashed line* in caudal cross section). Severing of sensory fibers at the epicenter causes axonal dieback caudal to the injury site (*red dashed line* in caudal section). As the injury progresses over several weeks, hemorrhaging and edema come to an end and microglia/macrophages phagocytose the cell and hemorrhagic debris. Oligodendrocytes undergo apoptotic cell death due to inflammation and white matter excitotoxicity, contributing to demyelination. Depending on the extent of damage to the meninges, fibroblasts *(orange)* proliferate and infiltrate the spinal cord, contributing to extracellular matrix (ECM) remodeling. Astrocytes proliferate, acting to seal off the injury, forming a glial scar *(black outline of cavity)*. Macrophages continue to infiltrate and phagocytose debris. At the level of injury, the majority of sensory and motor neurons are gone. Severed motor, sensory, and autonomic axons moving above and below the injury site have their distal ends (relative to the cell body) degraded, and the proximal ends retract. Angiogenesis also occurs (not shown). **(d)** Intermediate/chronic. The remaining debris is cleared from the lesion and microglia/macrophages remain active, contributing to neuropathic pain. Growth cones of regenerating sensory and motor neurons *(dashed lines)* meet either a physical barrier in the glial scar or an inhibitory chemical signal in the fibrous scar (due to chondroitin sulfate proteoglycans and myelin-associated proteins). Note that a subpial rim of surviving tissue exists in varying states of demyelination, representing a possible therapeutic target. In the lesion, macrophages, vascular-glial bundles, and astrocytes and collagenous fibers can be found. Remyelination is possible via either Schwann cells or oligodendrocyte precursor cells (OPCs). The time windows are largely based on preclinical studies in rodent models. It has been estimated that in humans the acute injury lasts up to 2 weeks, the subacute injury extends from 2 weeks to 6 months, and the chronic injury extends beyond the period of 6 months. (Reproduced from Austin J, Rowland J, Fehlings M. Pathophysiology of spinal cord injury. In: Fehlings M, Vaccaro A, Boakye M, Rossignol S, Ditunno J, Burns A, eds. Essentials of Spinal Cord Injury. New York: Thieme; 2013:44–45.)

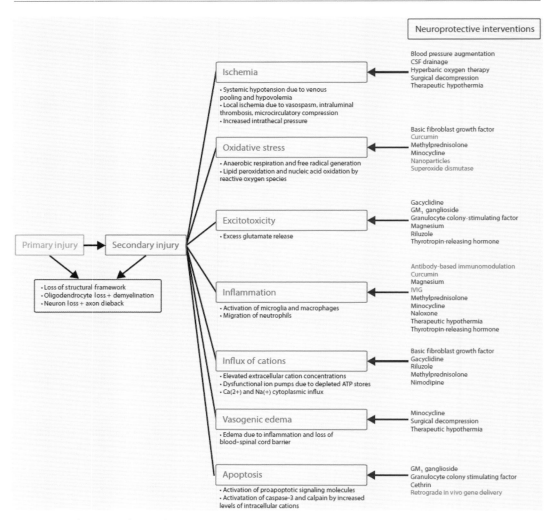

Fig. 8.2 Mechanisms of secondary injury after acute traumatic spinal cord injury. Potential neuroprotective strategies in clinical or preclinical trials are included with indication of their purported mechanisms of action. Interventions in blue have seen clinical trial, interventions in green are promising preclinical strategies. For illustrative purposes the complex interplay of these processes and their cascade of mediators have been omitted. ATP, adenosine triphosphate; CSF, cerebrospinal; IVIG, intravenous immunoglobulin G.

Table 8.1 Clinically Relevant Trials of Neuroprotective Interventions for Acute Spinal Cord Injury

Intervention	Purported Mechanism of Action	Trial Name	Participants (N)	Groups	Year Completed	Conclusions
Nonpharmacological						
MAP ≥ 85 mm Hg	Increases cord perfusion pressure by maintaining systemic blood pressure	MAPS	100	MAP ≥ 85 mm Hg × 7 days; MAP ≥ 65 mm Hg × 7 days	2017[†]	N/A
Surgical decompression	Mechanical decompression of the cord to improve microvascular circulation and alleviate pressure on cells	STASCIS	313	Early surgery (< 24 hours); late surgery (> 24 hours)	2012	ASIA motor improvement of two or more grades seen in 19.8% of early surgery group versus 8.8% in late surgery group
Pharmacological (phase III trials)						
MPSS	Interferes with inflammatory cytokines, attenuates peroxidation of neuronal membranes, and upregulates transcription of anti-inflammatory enzymes	NASCIS II	487	MPSS (30 mg/kg bolus then 5.4 mg/kg/h × 23 hours); naloxone (5.4 mg/kg bolus then 4.5 mg/kg/h × 23 hours); placebo	1990	No significant difference between groups; post hoc analysis revealed improved motor recovery with MPSS given within 8 hours of injury
		NASCIS III	499	MPSS (5.4 mg/kg/h × 24 hours); MPSS (5.4 mg/kg/h × 48 hours); tirilazad (2.5 mg/kg q6h × 48 hours)	1997	No significant difference between groups; post hoc analysis demonstrated improved motor scores with 48 hours MPSS regimen given between 3 and 8 hours after injury
Minocycline	Inhibits microglial activation and transcription of proinflammatory proteins such as COX-2, TNF-α, and IL-1β	MASC	248[*]	Minocycline (q12h decreasing doses of 800 mg, 700 mg, 600 mg, 500 mg, then 400 mg BID × 5 days); placebo	2018[†]	N/A
Naloxone	Suppresses microglial activation and the release of proinflammatory TNF-α, IL-1β, and neurotoxic superoxide free radicals	NASCIS II	487	MPSS (30 mg/kg bolus then 5.4 mg/kg/hr × 23 hours); naloxone (5.4 mg/kg bolus then 4.5 mg/kg/h × 23 hours); placebo	1990	No significant difference between groups

(continued)

Table 8.1 (*continued*)

Intervention	Purported Mechanism of Action	Trial Name	Participants (N)	Groups	Year Completed	Conclusions
Riluzole	Anti-excitotoxic, sodium-channel blocker, may inhibit presynaptic glutamate release and stimulate reuptake	RISCIS	351*	Riluzole (100 mg BID × 24 hours then 50 mg BID × 13 days); placebo	2017†	N/A
Cethrin	Inactivation of the Rho-ROCK pathway	Cethrin in Acute Cervical Spinal Cord Injury	N/A	High-dose Cethrin; low-dose Cethrin; placebo	2016†	N/A
Nimodipine	Calcium channel blocker that inhibits influx of calcium and activation of calcium-dependent processes (e.g., apoptotic enzyme activity, neurotransmitter release)	Pharmacological therapy of spinal cord injury during the acute phase	100	Nimodipine (0.015 mg/kg/h × 2 hours then 0.03 mg/kg/h × 7 days); MPSS (30 mg/kg bolus then 5.4 mg/kg/h × 23 hours); nimodipine + MPSS; placebo	1998	No significant difference between groups
Tirilazad mesylate	Inhibits neuronal membrane peroxidation	NASCIS III	499	MPSS (5.4 mg/kg/h × 24 hours); MPSS (5.4 mg/kg/h × 48 hours); tirilazad (2.5 mg/kg q6h × 48 hours)	1997	No significant difference between groups
GM₁-ganglioside	Activates neurotrophic factor receptor tyrosine kinases to influence neural plasticity, survival and repair	Sygen multi-center acute spinal cord injury study	797	Sygen (300 mg bolus then 100 mg/d × 56 days); sygen (600 mg bolus then 200 mg/d × 56 days); placebo	2001	No significant difference between groups

Abbreviations: ASIA, American Spinal Injury Association; BID, twice daily; COX, cyclooxygenase; GM-1, monosialotetrahexosylganglioside; IL, interleukin; MAP, mean arterial pressure; MAPS, Mean Arterial Blood Pressure Treatment for Acute Spinal Cord Injury; MASC, Minocycline in Acute Spinal Cord Injury; MPSS, methylprednisolone sodium succinate; N/A, not available; NASCIS, National Acute Spinal Cord Injury Study; RISCIS, Riluzole in Spinal Cord Injury Study; STASCIS, Surgical Timing in Acute Spinal Cord Injury Study; TNF, tumor necrosis factor.

*Projected enrollment as per https://www.clinicaltrials.gov.

†Project study completion date.

■ Ongoing and Completed Clinical Trials

Surgical Decompression

Cord edema, vertebral column deformity, and mechanical instability lead to ongoing cord compression and repeated insults after the primary injury. As a result, surgical intervention to decompress and stabilize the spine is critical in the acute setting. Multiple preclinical studies have demonstrated greater cell survival and improved behavioral outcomes with early versus late decompression. In 2012, the Surgical Treatment of Acute Spinal Cord Injury Study (STASCIS), a prospective, multicenter, cohort study of 313 patients, was published. It assessed outcome differences between early surgery (within 24 hours of injury; n = 182) and late surgery (> 24 hours; n = 131); a total of 222 patients were available for 6-month follow-up. Of the early decompression group, 19.8% demonstrated an improvement of two or more grades in the American Spinal Injury Association (ASIA) Impairment Scale (AIS) compared with 8.8% in the late decompression group.[1] A prospective cohort study of patients undergoing early (≤ 24 hours; n = 35) versus late (> 24 hours; n = 49) surgery for acute SCI was also published in 2012. At discharge from the rehabilitation facility, 27% of the early surgery group versus 3% of the late surgery group had improved by at least two AIS grades.[2] Furthermore, a 2015 observational cohort study involving 450 patients found that AIS grade B/C/D patients who had surgery within 24 hours recovered by 6.3 ASIA motor points more than those with surgery after 24 hours.[3] These studies together have provided evidence in favor of early surgical decompression.

Further clinical trials are underway to determine the ideal timing of surgery and to confirm results in other populations. AOSpine Europe is conducting a multicenter, prospective, observational study of early (≤ 12 hours) versus late (> 12 hours and < 14 days) decompression estimated to end in March 2017. The Optimal Treatment for Spinal Cord Injury Associated with Cervical Canal Stenosis (OSCIS) study is a randomized trial at Tokyo University exploring early (< 24 hours) versus delayed (> 14 days) surgery for acute cervical cord injury without bony injury. This study is restricted to ASIA grade C patients and is expected to conclude in December 2018.[4] See Chapter 6 for a more detailed discussion of surgical intervention.

Blood Pressure Augmentation

Acute spinal cord injuries can result in disruption of autonomic pathways and a loss of sympathetic tone below the level injury. A resultant decrease in venous return occurs due to redistribution of blood into the dependent atonic vasculature. The physiological compensatory mechanisms to maintain systemic perfusion are cardiac inotropy and chronotropy; however, these reflexes may be lost in cervical or high-thoracic injuries. In severe circumstances, life-threatening neurogenic shock may occur. This is particularly important in patients with multi-system trauma, in which vascular injuries and hypovolemia are common.

Systemic hypotension is associated with worse outcomes after many types of traumatic injury. Preclinical data demonstrate that even short periods of hypotension result in worsened neurologic outcomes after traumatic brain injury (TBI) and SCI. Although the normal spinal cord maintains perfusion pressure by autoregulatory mechanisms in a similar fashion to the brain, severe injury can induce vasospasm, intraluminal thrombosis, and microvascular compression. The result is a cord with compromised autoregulatory mechanisms that is highly vulnerable to systemic hypotension.[5]

Multiple prospective and retrospective clinical studies of blood pressure augmentation have been completed, providing a set of level III evidence in favor of elevated mean arterial pressure (MAP) targets as a preventative measure in SCI. Several studies in the 1990s demonstrated improved ASIA grades and outcome scores at follow-up in patients with target MAP ≥ 85 or 90 mm Hg immediately postinjury. The literature also suggests no significant increase in adverse events association with blood pressure augmentation. The American Association of Neurological Surgeons (AANS) and Congress of Neurological Surgeons (CNS) currently provide level III recommendations to correct hypotension (systolic blood pressure < 90 mm Hg) as soon as possible and maintain MAP at 85 to 90 mm Hg for the first 7 days following injury to improve cord perfusion.[6] This is commonly employed in clinical practice, but the optimal target pressure and duration of treatment continues to be explored.

Steroids

Methylprednisolone sodium succinate (MPSS) is a potent synthetic glucocorticoid that can bind cytoplasmic receptors with high affinity to interfere with inflammatory cytokines, arachidonic acid metabolites, and adhesion molecules, and upregulate the transcription of anti-inflammatory enzymes. In preclinical models of SCI, MPSS is also protective against oxidative stress and is associated with increased numbers of surviving oligodendrocytes and motor neurons. The successful clinical application of MPSS to autoimmune and other inflammatory conditions has led to a series of clinical trials for SCI over the last three decades.[7]

Although previous AANS/CNS guidelines recommended MPSS as a treatment option for SCI, the most recent iteration has dramatically revised this stance and provides level I recommendations against the administration of MPSS despite no new randomized controlled trial (RCT) data.[6] Here we summarize the cornerstone trials that have evaluated MPSS for acute SCI and underscore the importance of careful interpretation of the results in the context of a heterogeneous SCI population. Multiple observational studies have also been completed encompassing several thousand patients. Their results are varied, likely owing to a diverse patient population, differences in the pathophysiological basis of thoracic and cervical injuries, and the timing of interventions.

The National Acute Spinal Cord Injury Study (NASCIS), published in 1984, was a multicenter, prospective, double-blind, randomized trial (N = 330) of low-dose (100 mg bolus + 25 mg every 6 hours) versus high-dose (1,000 mg bolus + 250 mg every 6 hours) MPSS for 10 days. No significant differences in neurologic

outcome were found between dosing groups, but subsequent animal studies found that the high-dose regimen likely resulted in inadequate peak serum concentrations to have a neuroprotective effect.[8]

NASCIS II, published in 1990, was a randomized trial (N = 487) of high-dose MPSS for 1 day versus naloxone (5.4 mg/kg bolus and then 4.5 mg/kg/h for 23 hours) versus placebo. Although no difference was observed in motor scores, a significant improvement in light touch and pinprick sensation was found in the MPSS group. A priori, the authors had theorized that early drug administration would improve efficacy. A post hoc analysis, using the mode intervention time of 8 hours as a cutoff, demonstrated a significant improvement in sensory and motor scores with early initiation of therapy (within 8 hours of injury).[9] Although multiple subsequent RCTs attempted to validate this finding, they were plagued by methodological concerns that resulted in these positive findings being neither confirmed nor refuted.[7]

After parallel preclinical work better established the temporality of secondary injury, NASCIS III (published 1997; N = 499) was developed to explore a longer duration of treatment. This international, double-blind, randomized trial divided patients into short duration MPSS (30 mg/kg bolus and then 5.4 mg/kg/h for 24 hours), longer duration MPSS (30 mg/kg bolus and then 5.4 mg/kg/h for 48 hours) and tirilazad (2.5 mg/kg q6h for 48 hours) groups. The 48-hour MPSS group showed a trend toward greater motor improvement but had a higher rate of severe pneumonia and sepsis. A secondary analysis of time-to-treatment again used the mode intervention time as a cutoff (3 hours). The subset of 48-hour dosing MPSS patients who received therapy within 3 to 8 hours had significant improvements in motor scores over the 24-hour MPSS group.[10] A 2012 Cochrane review pooled data from multiple previous RCTs into a meta-analysis representing the highest quality evidence available on this topic. The data showed that NASCIS II MPSS dosing administered within 8 hours was associated with a four-point greater recovery at ≥ 6-month follow-up and, interestingly, a trend toward lower mortality.[11] This meta-analysis was not included in the 2013 AANS/CNS SCI guidelines despite its high quality and the clinically relevant conclusions.[6] For a more detailed discussion of MPSS for acute SCI, see Chapter 7.

Therapeutic Hypothermia

Therapeutic hypothermia has shown clinical utility as a neuroprotective strategy after cardiac arrest and other forms of hypoxic-ischemic encephalopathy. Cooling techniques include chilled intravenous fluids, surface cooling (e.g., cold packs, water-circulating blanket, air-circulating blanket, etc.), and intravascular catheter cooling. Managing a patient's response to cooling, such as shivering, vasoconstriction, coagulopathy, arrhythmias, and pain, is critical for safe, rapid, and sustainable cooling. A trained intensive care unit staff that is familiar with therapeutic hypothermia can provide appropriate sedation, analgesia, paralytics, and core temperature monitoring, and can manage the complications of cooling.

The physiological effect of cooling is a decrease in the basal metabolic rate of all tissues at a cellular level via slowed passive diffusion of molecules and dramatically reduced enzyme-catalyzed reaction rates. As a result, significant reductions are demonstrated in oxygen and glucose consumption, central nervous system (CNS) blood flow, neuroinflammation, apoptosis, free radical generation (superoxide, peroxynitrite, hydrogen peroxide), thromboxane A_2 levels, and CNS–blood barrier permeability. Clinical trials have shown a decrease in O_2 consumption and CO_2 production of 6 to 10% per degree Celsius (25 to 40% at 33°C in humans).[12,13] These promising effects have led to the launch of numerous clinical trials of hypothermia for various forms of CNS protection. Its application to SCI is a logical step, and it has now been extensively studied in animal models. A recent meta-analysis of 16 preclinical studies showed improvements in behavioral outcomes by ~ 25% for both systemic and regional hypothermia, although heterogeneity between studies was notably high.[13]

These promising data led the Miami Project to Cure Paralysis group in 2009 to complete a pilot study prospectively assessing systemic hypothermia for acute SCI. This study of 14 patients showed a trend toward improved functional outcomes at 1 year without an increase in adverse events.[14] The next generation of this trial, pending approval, is the Acute Rapid Cooling Therapy for Injuries of the Spinal Cord (ARCTIC), which is a phase II/III clinical trial of 200 patients with cooling initiated within 6 hours of injury.[4] It is hoped that this larger trial will answer questions regarding short- and long-term clinical efficacy and the risks of systemic hypothermia in trauma patients.

Therapeutic hypothermia has had success in CNS protection after cardiac arrest through careful patient selection and intervention monitoring. If used judiciously, and in the appropriate population, therapeutic hypothermia could become a valuable neuroprotective adjunct for SCI in the future.

Riluzole

Riluzole is an oral, U.S. Food and Drug Administration (FDA)-approved, benzothiazole antiepileptic used in amyotrophic lateral sclerosis (ALS) to delay ventilator-dependence and increase survival. Riluzole antagonizes tetrodotoxin-sensitive sodium channels found on injured neurons. It may also inhibit presynaptic glutamate release and stimulate reuptake to accelerate clearance. Together, these effects are thought to be neuroprotective against excitotoxicity and apoptosis. In preclinical models of SCI, it has demonstrated improved behavioral outcomes with larger populations of surviving neurons.

The North American Clinical Trials Network (NACTN) conducted a phase I safety study in 2014 of riluzole for SCI. Adverse events were not higher in the treatment group. The study found that patients with complete injuries (ASIA grade A) treated with riluzole were twice as likely to convert to incomplete injury (ASIA B or better)—50% versus 24% conversion at 90 days.[15] Based on these exciting results, the NACTN has now launched a phase II/III RCT, the Riluzole in Spinal Cord Injury Study (RISCIS), which will include 350 patients assessed by the ASIA scale, the Spinal Cord Independence Measure (SCIM), the and Brief Pain Inventory.[4]

Minocycline

Minocycline is a highly lipid-soluble tetracycline antibiotic, giving it the greatest CNS penetration of its class. Minocycline inhibits microglial activation and transcription of important proinflammatory proteins such as cyclooxygenase-2 (COX-2), tumor necrosis factor-α (TNF-α), and interleukin-1β (IL-1β). Animal studies have demonstrated that application of minocycline results in reduced oligodendrocyte and neuron apoptosis, decreased lesion size, reduced inflammation, and improved behavioral outcomes.

These exciting results led to a phase II single-center, double-blind, randomized trial being published in 2012. This study compared 7 days of intravenous minocycline (n = 27) versus placebo (n = 25) in acute SCI, with confirmation of both serum and cerebrospinal fluid (CSF) steady-state drug levels. The trial demonstrated the safety of IV minocycline administration for SCI. Although not statistically significant, a trend toward improved motor scores was found.[16] This has led to the Minocycline in Acute Spinal Cord Injury (MASC) phase III clinical trial, which is expected to conclude in June 2018. This trial will compare 7 days of minocycline (started within 12 hours of injury) versus placebo and will compare multiple clinical outcome measures.[4]

Cethrin

Rho is a small guanosine triphosphatase (GTPase) with multiple downstream targets including Rho kinase (ROCK). Rho is a potent inhibitor of cytoskeletal growth and cell motility, it and plays a key role in the post-SCI apoptosis cascade. Via ROCK it also induces neuron retraction and growth cone collapse. Cethrin is a recombinant variant of C3 transferase, a protein subunit of botulinum toxin, which locks Rho in the inactive state. When administered intraoperatively on the dura in a fibrin sealant carrier, it has been shown to decrease lesion size, enhance cellular regeneration, and improve behavioral outcomes.[17]

A phase I/IIa study of Cethrin (N = 48) completed in 2011 was designed as a dose-finding study with incremental increases from 0.3 mg to 9 mg. No serious adverse events attributable to the drug were reported. Overall, 31% of the cervical patients and 66% of the 3-mg cervical cohort converted from ASIA A to ASIA C or D.[17] This exciting result led to a phase II/III double-blind, randomized, multicenter trial of Cethrin that is scheduled to begin this year (2016). The study design will assign ASIA grade A or B patients with C4–C6 level injuries to low-dose Cethrin, high-dose Cethrin, or placebo. Outcome measures will include the ASIA scale, the SCIM III, and the Graded Redefined Assessment of Strength, Sensibility and Prehension (GRASSP).[4]

Thyrotropin-Releasing Hormone

Thyrotropin-releasing hormone (TRH) is a tripeptide hormone produced in the paraventricular nuclei of the hypothalamus. TRH is a key component of hypothalamic-pituitary homeostatic mechanisms and possesses potent analeptic properties. Its neuroprotective effects stem from antagonization of platelet-activating factor (PAF), excitotoxin, and peptidoleukotriene effects in the postinjury environment.

In preclinical testing, TRH has demonstrated improvement of long-term motor outcomes in TBI and SCI. In 1995, a phase II, double-blind, randomized clinical trial in SCI (N = 20) was completed showing significant gains in motor, sensory, and overall neurologic injury (Sunnybrook Cord Injury Scale) scores for incomplete injuries (n = 6).[18] However, the results must be interpreted carefully, as many patients were lost to follow-up from already small experimental groups. No other trials of TRH for SCI have been registered or reported. The initial success in pilot testing suggests a larger trial may be of benefit.

Cerebrospinal Fluid Drainage

Postinjury spinal cord ischemia can result in significantly increased cell death and neurologic disability. Spinal cord blood flow is a function of inflow arterial pressure, outflow venous pressure, and intrathecal pressure. Elevation of MAP generates greater inflow forces, whereas CSF drainage decreases intrathecal pressure (ITP) and compression of the vasculature. Both of these measures attempt to prevent tissue hypoperfusion in the critical postinjury period.

The CSF drainage for reduction of ITP has a clinical precedent in aortic aneurysm surgery, where prophylactic drainage can help to decrease the risk of cord ischemia and postoperative neurologic deficits. Completed in 2009, a phase I/II RCT of 22 patients with acute SCI found that CSF drainage alone was not associated with any improvement in outcomes or adverse effects.[19] This study, however, was underpowered and thus was unable to demonstrate efficacy.

A recent experiment in a porcine SCI model demonstrated a 24% increase in cord flow when using a combination of CSF drainage with MAP elevation.[20] Based on these promising results, a phase IIB randomized trial of CSF drainage in combination with MAP elevation after acute SCI was planned to start in August 2015. In this protocol, treatments begin during surgical decompression and continue for 5 days postinjury. The target intrathecal pressure is 10 mm Hg, and the target MAP is 100 to 110 mm Hg. Results are expected by December 2017.[4]

Fibroblast Growth Factor

The fibroblast growth factor (FGF) family consists of heparin-binding proteins that play a key role in mitogenesis, angiogenesis, embryonic development, wound healing, and tissue proliferation. Basic FGF has been used in preclinical models of Alzheimer's disease and Parkinson's disease to interrupt the excitotoxic neurodegenerative cascade by stabilizing intracellular calcium levels and suppressing oxyradical production. In multiple animal SCI models, basic FGF administration by intrathecal osmotic minipump has been shown to improve locomotion and respiratory function, and to enhance endogenous cell survival.[21] Based on these exciting results, a phase I/II multicenter, randomized, double-blind trial ($N = 164$) of an FGF analogue, SUN13837 (Asubio Pharmaceuticals Inc., Edison, NJ), has been initiated to assess safety and efficacy in ASIA A/B/C patients within 12 hours of injury. The study has completed, with results expected in 2016.[4]

Hepatocyte Growth Factor

Hepatocyte growth factor (HGF) is a ligand for the c-Met receptor that promotes mature hepatocyte mitogenesis and hepatic angiogenesis and increases cell motility. Human HGF plasmid DNA therapy is being trialed in completed myocardial infarction and the ongoing ischemia of coronary artery disease to improve angiogenesis and protect cardiomyocytes. Recent evidence demonstrates that HGF may also have utility in CNS protection. HGF applied to models of stroke has been shown to enhance microcirculation through angiogenesis and to prevent degradation of the blood–brain barrier, leading to protection from secondary injury after an ischemic event.[22,23]

This finding has been adapted to SCI models, showing that exogenous administration of HGF promotes survival of neurons and oligodendrocytes and improves behavioral outcomes. Moreover, in animals receiving intrathecal HGF, the gross cavitation area at the injury site was reduced, the number of motor neurons in the ventral horns was increased, and caspase-3 (apoptosis-mediator) activation was inhibited.[23] Recombinant human HGF has been shown to promote angiogenesis and improve upper limb function in nonhuman primate cervical cord injury models, which is an important proof-of-concept step in preclinical trials.[22]

A phase I clinical trial of intrathecal recombinant human HGF for SCI has now begun, with completion scheduled for 2017.[4]

Hyperbaric Oxygen Therapy

Systemic hypoperfusion, microvascular compression, and loss of autoregulatory mechanisms are important factors leading to ischemic secondary injury. Tissue hypoxia triggers inefficient anaerobic respiration and leads to increased superoxide, hydrogen peroxide, and nitric oxide levels. These molecules cause oxidative damage to lipids, proteins, and DNA, further contributing to the secondary injury. Nitric oxide also plays a key role in vascular tone, neuronal communication, and thrombocyte function.

Hyperbaric oxygen (HBO) therapy has patients breathe 100% oxygen in a hyperbaric chamber pressurized to 2 to 3 atmospheres. It results in a shift of the alveolar-capillary oxygen absorption equation and increased partial pressures of oxygen in all body tissues. Theoretically, this improved oxygen delivery in the microcirculation can reduce ischemia and help to maintain aerobic metabolism. Additionally, nitric oxide can be cleared by oxidization with oxygen to nitrite (NO^{-2}) and nitrate (NO^{-3}). Furthermore, HBO therapy has been shown to increase levels of antioxidant enzymes superoxide dismutase (SOD) and catalase, which scavenge free radicals.[24]

Preclinical studies have shown improved motor scores and a greater numbers of surviving neurons in the cords of animals treated with HBO therapy either very early (< 4 hours) or early (4 hours to < 24 hours). On histopathological examination, decreased necrotic tissue volume, hemorrhage, and markers of inflammation were found with HBO treatment. Few clinical trials of HBO for SCI have been reported owing to the logistical difficulties in applying HBO therapy to critically ill multisystem trauma patients and the costs of treatment. Several small studies were published in the 1980s suggesting a possible benefit to HBO therapy. In 2000, a retrospective study of 34 patients with hyperextension cervical spinal cord injuries found that those who received HBO therapy have marginally better outcomes, but this may have been a function of patient selection for each group (i.e., patients with a lower severity of injury were candidates for HBO therapy). No further studies of HBO for SCI have been registered or reported.[25]

Granulocyte Colony-Stimulating Factor

Granulocyte colony-stimulating factor (G-CSF) is a glycoprotein that functions as a cytokine and hormone to stimulate the bone marrow production of granulocytes. It also stimulates the proliferation, differentiation, and survival of mature neutrophils and their precursors.

Recent evidence shows that G-CSF can enhance survival of ischemic cells in the myocardium and CNS. Moreover, G-CSF receptors have been found in the brain and spinal cord, where it acts as a neurotrophic factor promoting neurogenesis and protecting against glutamate-induced apoptosis. These properties have resulted in successful preclinical and early-phase clinical trials of G-CSF for CNS insults such as stroke. This work has been further extended to preclinical trials in rodent models of SCI.

Experiments in vivo have demonstrated significantly increased numbers of surviving neurons in the injured spinal cords of mice treated with exogenous G-CSF. Immunohistochemistry analyses have revealed diminished neuronal apoptotic events in treated mice and reduced expression of inflammatory cytokines IL-1β and TNF-α. Furthermore, the myelinated white matter tracts of injured cords were larger and contained greater numbers of oligodendrocytes expressing antiapoptotic Bcl-Xl protein. Most importantly, these changes resulted in improved motor scores and qualitative function.

Translational application of G-CSF to SCI trials may be more readily performed than with other drugs. It has already been shown to be safe in active clinical use for hematopoietic stimulation during chemotherapy, and is actively being trialed in ischemic stroke. A phase I/IIa trial completed in 2012 compared low-dose G-CSF (5 µg/kg/d for 5 days) with high-dose G-CSF (10 µg/kg/d for 5 days) for safety and efficacy. AIS scores improved after both low- and high-dose G-CSF administration and to a greater extent in the high-dose group. No serious adverse events were encountered in the study. It is important to note, however, that this study lacked an appropriate control and had inherent selection biases.[26] In 2015, another phase I/IIa trial of 10 µg/kg/d × 5 days G-CSF ($n = 28$) was compared with high-dose NASCIS II protocol MPSS ($n = 34$). Of the G-CSF group patients with AIS grade B or C (incomplete injuries), 17.9% improved by two or more grades compared with no patients in the MPSS group.[27] It will be important for future trials to address efficacy in a prospective, randomized, placebo-controlled fashion. The appropriate therapeutic window also requires further exploration.

Magnesium

N-methyl-D-aspartic acid (NMDA) and non-NMDA receptors play a key role by binding to excitatory amino acids in the excitotoxic-apoptotic cascade. Neutrophil infiltration has also been implicated in the secondary destruction of surviving cells and the neural architecture. Magnesium (Mg) is an extensively studied NMDA receptor antagonist that has demonstrated antiapoptotic properties in experimental models of TBI, myocardial infarction, and organ transplant. In rodent models of SCI it has shown neuroprotective properties leading to decreased neutrophil infiltration, increased oligodendrocyte survival, and improved behavioral outcomes. This is particularly true when administered within 4 hours of injury, resulting in reduced lesion sizes and further improvements in motor function at several months.[28]

Although intravenous Mg chloride and Mg sulfate preparations are commonly used in the clinical setting as Mg^{2+} replacements, CNS concentrations are not affected significantly enough to be neuroprotective. Combining magnesium chloride with an excipient, polyethylene glycol (PEG 3350) has been shown to increase CNS Mg concentrations more effectively in rat models. A phase II, double-blind, randomized, placebo-controlled trial ($N = 16$) of pegylated magnesium (q6h × 6 doses) versus placebo in ASIA A/B/C patients treated within 12 hours has completed, with results expected in 2016.

Naloxone

Naloxone is a competitive opioid receptor antagonist commonly used to reverse CNS depression by opioid overdose. In preclinical experiments it has been shown to suppress microglial activation and the subsequent release of proinflammatory TNF-α, IL-1β, and neurotoxic superoxide free radicals. A phase I clinical trial published in 1985 found some improvement in neurologic function and somatosensory evoked potentials after naloxone administration.[29] In 1990, NASCIS II completed a randomized, double-blind, multicenter trial of methylprednisolone ($n = 162$) versus naloxone ($n = 154$) versus placebo ($n = 171$). Naloxone was not associated with any improvement in neurologic outcomes after acute SCI.[9] No further trials of naloxone have been registered or reported.

Gacyclidine

Glutamate-mediated excitotoxicity is an important cause of neuronal loss following traumatic cord injuries. Gacyclidine is a noncompetitive NMDA receptor antagonist that blocks receptor activation sites to reduce the excitotoxic influx of calcium that occurs with excess extracellular glutamate.

A phase II clinical trial was completed in 1999 that compared three doses of gacyclidine with a placebo ($N = 280$).[30] No significant differences in outcome were found between groups, and further clinical trials of gacyclidine in SCI have not been registered or reported.

Nimodipine

Nimodipine is a dihydropyridine calcium channel blocker commonly used to prevent vasospasm in subarachnoid hemorrhage. Calcium channel blockade could potentially reduce the influx of cations in the excitotoxic cascade. A phase III RCT ($N = 100$), completed in 1998, failed to demonstrate any significant difference in outcomes with nimodipine alone or in combination with methylprednisolone.[30] No further clinical trials of nimodipine for SCI have been published.

GM$_1$-Ganglioside

Monosialotetrahexosylganglioside (GM_1)-ganglioside is a glycosphingolipid present in the cell membranes of CNS cells. GM_1 has important effects on neural plasticity, survival, and repair by activating neurotrophic factor receptor tyrosine kinases. This effect is synergistic in the presence of neural growth factors and has been exploited successfully in multiple preclinical trials for Parkinson's disease, stroke, and Huntington's disease. A 1991 phase II randomized trial of GM_1 for SCI ($N = 37$) demonstrated enhanced ASIA motor scores at 1 year in patients treated with GM_1 sodium salt daily for 18 to 32 days.[31] This prompted the 2001 Sygen Multicenter Acute Spinal Cord Injury Study, a phase III randomized, double-blind, multicenter trial ($N = 797$) that showed a non-significant trend toward improved motor and sensory scores with GM_1 administration.[32] No further studies of GM_1 for SCI have been undertaken. The AANS/CNS currently provide level I recommendations against GM_1-ganglioside use in the treatment of acute SCI.

▓ Preclinical Studies

Antibody-Based Immunomodulation

The inflammatory cascade following SCI is a complex interplay of inflammatory cells, cytokine signaling, and cellular debris. Of particular interest are the divergent populations of activated (M1) and alternatively activated (M2) macrophages that can be beneficial to cell survival by phagocytosing debris and cellular remnants, and detrimental to cell survival by promoting excessive inflammatory response and axonal dieback. M2 macrophages, in particular, have efficient lysosomes and increased phagocytic activity to remove glial scar and cellular debris. IL-6 is an important trigger of the inflammatory response after SCI, upregulating the expression of inflammatory cytokines. Temporally controlled anti–IL-6 receptor antibody treatment has been shown to improve locomotor recovery in rats following contusive SCI. The pathophysiological basis of this recovery in part may be attributable to disproportionate differentiation of macrophages into M1 (decreased) and M2 (increased) populations at the lesion site. Other important effects of anti–IL-6 receptor antibody treatment include decreased TNF-α expression and diminished migration of neutrophils to the injured cord.[33]

Antibody-based immunomodulation of interleukins, or other signaling molecules, forms an important field for future research. Additionally, given the vast number of targets available, this therapeutic strategy holds the potential for exciting discoveries over the next decade.

Intravenous Immunoglobulin G

Intravenous immunoglobulin G (IVIG) is a pooled blood product of extracted immunoglobulin G (IgG) antibodies acquired from thousands of donors. IVIG has been used to successfully and safely attenuate the inflammatory cascade in multiple neurologic autoimmune conditions such as Guillain-Barré syndrome and chronic inflammatory demyelinating polyneuropathy. It also has been applied to rodent cervical models of SCI, where it was associated with reduced neutrophil infiltration at the injury site and decreased levels of proinflammatory cytokines IL-1β, IL-6, and chemokine monocyte chemoattractant protein-1 (MCP-1). Rats treated with IVIG also displayed improved locomotion, hind-limb function, and electrophysiological recordings of axonal conduction.[34]

Although the mechanisms of action in SCI continue to be elucidated, recent work suggests IVIG may attenuate neutrophil infiltration by interfering with adhesion and inducing neutrophil apoptosis. Other mechanisms may include modulation of Fcγ receptors, which are important for phagocytosis, and scavenging of activated complement system fragments. These multiple mechanisms of immunomodulation, the successful early SCI studies, and decades of clinical experience make IVIG an attractive neuroprotective agent for future translation. First, however, the dose range and therapeutic window must be established in preclinical models. Second, a more detailed understanding of the mechanisms of action in SCI are needed before moving toward translation.[35]

Nanoparticles

Nanoparticles are uniform particles of any material between 1 and 100 nanometers in size. They can be reactants themselves or can be bound to various drugs, enzymes, antibodies, and fluorescent dyes. Although multiple molecules discussed in this chapter have been successfully delivered using nanoparticle vehicles (e.g., MPSS, minocycline, DNA plasmids, neuro-

9

Hydrogel Biomaterials in Spinal Cord Repair and Regeneration

Manuel Ingo Günther, Thomas Schackel, Norbert Weidner, and Armin Blesch

▪ Introduction

Due to the limited regeneration of the adult mammalian spinal cord, injuries lead to mostly irreversible damage and functional deterioration. Effective means to promote repair of the damaged spinal cord do not exist, although considerable progress has been made in the past three decades. The loss of neurons and glia and the disruption of the descending, ascending, and intraspinal tracts contribute to motor, sensory, and autonomic deficits. Approaches to promote recovery after spinal cord injury (SCI) include the stimulation of the intrinsic regenerative capacity of injured neurons, neutralization of growth inhibitory factors, degradation of inhibitory extracellular matrix (ECM), modulation of inflammatory responses, and provision of axon growth-promoting molecules and substrates at the lesion site. The latter was initially focused on cell transplantation to provide a substrate for axons to extend across a lesion site, and substantial advances in identifying cells suitable to replace tissue lost at the lesion site have been made. However, several obstacles, including poor cell survival, a lack of rostrocaudally directed axon growth and guidance, potential immune responses to cell transplants, the risk of tumor formation, and regulatory hurdles for cell products, complicate the clinical translation of cell therapies. Therefore, an off-the-shelf product, such as biomaterials that can mimic at least some of the roles of trans-planted cells or improve the physiological influences of cells on axon regeneration, would be of high value. Transplantation of different materials that emulate cellular and extracellular properties to physically support endogenous cells and regenerating axons in a three-dimensional (3D) matrix has become an area of intense investigation. In addition, biomaterials can also be used as drug delivery devices to complement and enhance cell transplantation strategies (**Table 9.1**).

To successfully implement biomaterials in the injured spinal cord, several characteristics are particularly relevant. Materials should be biocompatible without toxicity or immunologic reaction to implants or degradation products that might induce fibroglial scarring and impede spinal cord regeneration. The implanted material should be able to fill cystic cavities, integrate into the surrounding host spinal cord, provide a permissive substrate for cells, and guide the growth of injured axons in a rostrocaudal direction to bridge a lesion gap. Support of host-derived or transplanted myelinating cells is another important requirement for the proper functioning of regenerating axons. The exchange of nutrients and oxygen with the surrounding parenchyma and, when larger scaffolds are used, neovascularization are key for the successful integration in the injured spinal cord. The sustained release of growth factors and neurotrophic factors by implanted materials would also be valuable in further enhancing

Table 9.1 Comparison of Different Properties of Hydrogel Biomaterials and Some Combinations of Other Treatments with Biomaterials

Name	Source	Chemical characteristics	Gel formation	Structure	Degra-dation	Combinatory strategies
PEG	Synthetic	Linear polyether	Copolymerization and chemical cross-linking	Anisotropic; channels	–	SCs
				Isotropic	+	NT-3, BDNF
pHEMA	Synthetic	Linear poly-methacrylate	Chemical cross-linking	Isotropic	–	bFGF, surface modification
				Anisotropic; conduit	–	Other biomaterials and trophic factors
pHPMA	Synthetic	Linear poly-methacrylate	Chemical cross-linking	Isotropic	–	Surface modification
PLA	Synthetic	Linear polyester	Salt leaching, CO_2 foaming, freeze-drying	Isotropic	+	OECs, NAs
				Anisotropic: micropores	+	Neurotrophic factors, SCs
				Anisotropic: microfiber sheets	–	Fibrin
				Anisotropic: conduit	–	SCs
PLGA	Synthetic	Linear polyester	Salt leaching, CO_2 foaming, freeze-drying	Isotropic	+	PLL, NSCs
				Anisotropic: channels	+	NSCs, SCs, gene delivery
Agarose	Natural (seaweed)	Linear poly-saccharide	Spontaneous, critical point drying, lyophilization	Isotropic	+	BDNF
				Isotropic	+	Methylprednisolone, ChABC, NT-3
				Anisotropic: channels	–	BDNF, BDNF- and NT-3 expressing BMSCs, viral vectors for NT-3
Alginate	Natural (seaweed)	Linear poly-saccharide	Ionotropic gelation, chemical cross-linking, penetrating polymer networks	Capsules	–	BDNF-expressing fibroblasts

Material	Source	Polymer type	Cross-linking method	Architecture		Additional components
Chitosan	Natural (crustaceans)	Linear polysaccharide	Chemical cross-linking, penetrating polymer networks	Isotropic	+	Fibrinogen, GDNF, VEGF
				Anisotropic: channels	–	NPCs, BDNF-expressing BMSCs
				Anisotropic: conduits	–/–	Peripheral nerve grafts, laminin coating + NPCs, fibrin/laminin + dibutyryl cAMP, NPCs + growth factor cocktail
Collagen	Natural (bone and cartilage)	Triple helix protein	Spontaneous, electro-spinning, chemical cross-linking	Isotropic	+	Laminin, SCs
				Anisotropic: aligned fibers	–	BDNF, EGFR-antibody
				Anisotropic: honeycombs	–	BMSCs
				Anisotropic: channels	–	
				Anisotropic: channels + aligned fibers	–	NT-3
Fibrin	Natural (fibrinogen/thrombin)	Coagulated protein fibers	Spontaneous gelation of fibrinogen fragments	Isotropic	+	ChABC; fibrinogen, NSCs, heparin + NT-3; heparin + NT-3 + PDGF + NPCs; peripheral nerve grafts + aFGF; aFGF
Hyaluronic acid	Natural (ECM)	Linear polysaccharide	Spontaneous, chemical modification/cross-linking	Isotropic	+	PDGF, NPCs
Matrigel	Natural (basement membrane proteins)	Protein mixture	Spontaneous	Isotropic	–	
				Isotropic	+	SCs
Self-assembling peptides	Synthesized	Defined peptide(s)	Spontaneous	Aligned fibers but macroscopically isotropic	+	NSCs

Abbreviations: aFGF, acidic fibroblast growth factor; BDNF, brain-derived neurotrophic factor; bFGF, basic fibroblast growth factor; BMSC, bone marrow stromal cell; cAMP, cyclic adenosine monophosphate; ChABC, chondroitinase ABC; ECM, extracellular matrix; EGFR, epidermal growth factor receptor; GDNF, glial cell line-derived neurotrophic factor; NA, neonatal astrocytes; NPC, neural progenitor cell; NSC, neural stem cell; NT-3, neurotrophin-3; OEC, olfactory ensheathing cells; PDGF, platelet-derived growth factor; PEG, polyethylene glycol pHEMA, poly(2-hydroxyethyl methacrylate); pHPMA, poly(2-hydroxypropyl methacrylamide); PLA, polylactic acid; PLGA, polylactic-co-glycolic acid; PLL, poly-L-lysine; SC, Schwann cells; VEGF, vascular endothelial growth factor.

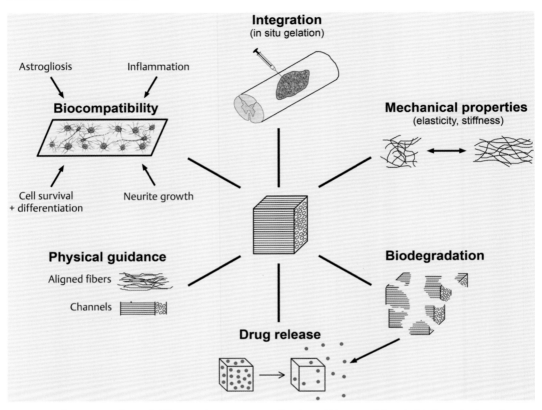

Fig. 9.1 Schematic outline of different characteristics of hydrogel biomaterials suitable for spinal cord repair.

axon growth and cell survival. Finally, noninvasive means to deliver biomaterials acquiring the final 3D structure in situ by self-assembly would be superior to implantation of a structure with predefined size and appearance, due to the irregular shape of spinal cord lesions (**Fig. 9.1**).

Although no single biomaterial available to date can fulfill all of these criteria, hydrogels have some intriguing features making them particularly well suited for applications in the nervous system. The wide variety of available materials to generate hydrogels, the possibility of modulating physical (e.g., stiffness, elasticity, orientation) and chemical (e.g., degradation, surface modification) parameters, and their high water content enable adjustments to be made to mimic key features of the spinal cord and its ECM. Indeed, the ECM of soft tissue is a natural hydrogel composed of a mix of pro-

teins, proteoglycans, and glycosaminoglycan macromolecules that are cross-linked in a 3D network with high water content. Thus, hydrogels that provide an ECM with chemical and biological cues that are conducive for cells and axons might be able to promote axon regeneration and functional recovery after SCI.

Advantages and General Properties of Hydrogels

Hydrogels represent a transition between liquids and solids and are elastic, coherent, colloid-dispersal systems consisting of one or more dispersed components and water. On a microscopic scale, gels are heterogeneous, but in most cases isotropic on a macroscopic scale. Common hydrogels often contain only very small amounts of the gelling agents (usually less than 2%) and consist primarily of water. The macroscopic structure, including pore size, and the mechanical properties, such as the elasticity of hydrogels, are determined by the concentration and the molecular weight of the polymer molecules and the number and rigidity of linkages between the polymers. Due to their hydrophilic nature, hydrogels exhibit low interfacial tensions and good tissue integration and enable cell migration, an advantage over other scaffold materials. In addition to the chemical and structural properties of hydrogels, modifications of the surface by coating with proteins and peptides can enhance biocompatibility and cell adhesion, and reduce immune response and scarring. Hydrogels may also be useful as a drug-release system from layer-by-layer coated hydrogels, micro/nanoparticles, or injectable hydrogels.

Gels derived from biological macromolecules commonly display higher biocompatibility compared with gels from synthetic polymers because they can have intrinsic bioactivities that can modulate cellular behavior. However, insufficient stability due to weak chemical bonds resulting in rapid biodegradation might require chemical stabilization of natural biomaterials. Studies of hydrogels in animal models of peripheral nervous system (PNS) regeneration have advanced more rapidly than applications in central nervous system (CNS) injuries, and several ongoing and completed clinical trials have used channels to reconnect transected nerve fibers.[1] In the injured spinal cord, biomaterials that provide only a substrate for axon growth are unlikely to restore function without any additional intervention. Unlike the PNS, the CNS has only a limited intrinsic capacity for regeneration, and the inhibitory environment in and around a spinal cord lesion and the lack of appropriate axon growth stimuli further restrict regeneration. Biomaterials are well suited to physically reconnect spinal cord stumps across cavities and intraparenchymal cysts. In-situ self-assembling hydrogels that are injected and gelatinize directly in the lesion site are ideal to fill irregular-shaped lesion cavities to serve as an artificial substrate for axon growth. However, such hydrogels as well

as many scaffolds that are gelatinized before implantation lack an anisotropic structure to guide axonal regeneration.

Based on the chemical background of polymers, hydrogels can be divided into two broad categories: hydrogels made from synthetic polymers and those made from natural polymers. Each group can be further subdivided based on their chemical composition, modifications, or directional properties.

Hydrogels from Synthetic Polymers

One of the most important properties of hydrogels, especially for materials made from synthetic polymers, is their biocompatibility. The most common synthetic polymers for the formation of hydrogels that can be safely applied in vivo are based on poly(ethylene glycol), methacrylates, or aliphatic polyesters derived from lactide/glycolide.

Polyethylene Glycol

Polyethylene glycol (PEG) is a linear, liquid, hydrophilic polyether, and its viscosity depends on the chain length. Chemical alterations and cross-linking after functionalization of the terminal hydroxyl groups leads to the formation of a stable hydrogel with tunable properties such as permeability, molecular diffusivity, water content, elasticity, and degradation rate. Due to its hydrophilic nature, PEG is a known fusogen and can repair mechanically injured cells by resealing the plasma membrane and protecting mitochondria. In a chronic spinal cord transection, PEG has been shown to improve axon regeneration, vascularization, and astrocyte and Schwann cell infiltration, and to enable small functional improvements.[2] Despite its positive effect on mechanically injured cells, liquid PEG cannot serve as a scaffold for structural support and has to be chemically modified and cross-linked to form a stable hydrogel matrix. However, covalently cross-linked oligo[poly(ethylene glycol) fumarate] scaffolds with channel structure fail to promote substantial axonal regeneration into a lesion, even when seeded with Schwann cells.[3] Functionalized PEG such as acrylated polylactic acid (PLA)-b-PEG-b-PLA macromere and injectable Poly(N-isopropylacrylamide)-g-polyethylene glycol hydrogel (PNIPAAm-g-PEG) have been used for growth factor release promoting modest recovery of locomotor function.[4] However, neuroprotection or collateral sprouting rather than axon regeneration seem to underlie these effects. Functionalization of PEG with peptides that enhance cell adhesion and axonal growth in vitro should be considered in future in vivo studies.

Poly(2-Hydroxyethyl Methacrylate) (pHEMA)and Poly(2-Hydroxypropyl Methacrylamide) (pHPMA)

Both pHEMA and pHPMA are linear hydrophilic polymers produced by the polymerization of 2-hydroxyethyl methacrylate and 2-hydroxypropyl methacrylamide, respectively. Porous biocompatible hydrogels that are not biodegradable can be produced by cross-linking, and their properties can be fine-tuned by copolymerization with other acrylic acid derivatives, changes in the cross-linking density, or chemical modification. Porous pHEMA hydrogels with mechanical properties similar to those of spinal cord tissue support angiogenesis and possibly reduce astrogliosis. However, unmodified pHEMA scaffolds have only minor potential as a substrate for axonal regeneration, even in combination with growth factors.

By copolymerization with other monomers, a positively charged pHEMA scaffold with superior properties can be produced, providing a matrix for blood vessels and axons. Heparin complexed basic fibroblast growth factor-2 (FGF-2), which can be electrostatically attached to the scaffolds, seems to enhance axon growth, blood vessel extension, and functional recovery without any histological proof for axon growth across the lesion.[5] pHEMA scaffolds have also been modified with different biomolecules, such as cholesterol-modified superporous pHEMA scaffolds with different elastic moduli, which demonstrate ingrowth of blood vessels, axons, and Schwann cells. In addition to porous sponges, pHEMA as well as poly(2-hydroxyethyl methacrylate-co-methyl methacrylate) (pHEMA-MMA) channels have been used to promote tissue reconstruction across large transections in combination with peripheral nerves, fibrin glue, and FGF-1/heparin. Filling pHEMA-MMA tubes with collagen, fibrin, matrigel, methylcellulose, or smaller pHEMA-MMA tubes in combination with growth factors (FGF-1 or neurotrophin-3 [NT-3]) results in increased axon density within the channel.[6] A cross-linked pHPMA scaffold with a highly porous structure is commercialized under the name NeuroGel™ (NeuroGel En Marche Association, Crolles, France) has mechanical properties similar to neural tissue and is stable in the injured spinal cord for up to 21 months.[7] After complete spinal cord transections in rats and cats, myelinated axons, blood vessels, and ECM are found in the grafted gel. However, there is no evidence of long-distance axon growth into or through the matrix.

Taken together, pHEMA implants seem to be insufficient to support seeded cells, angiogenesis, and axonal regeneration. Changing the physical characteristics by copolymerization, chemical modification, or combination with other materials may enhance its potential for future applications in SCI research. Porous pHPMA hydrogels have shown some potential, but available data indicate a modest increase in randomly oriented axon growth rather than axon regeneration across the implant. Significantly more data are needed to evaluate the value of these scaffolds for clinical applications.

Polylactic Acid (PLA) and Polylactic-Co-Glycolic Acid (PLGA)

Both PLA and PLGA, a copolymer of PLA and polyglycolic acid (PGA), are linear, aliphatic polyesters that are biodegradable and biocompatible. Highly porous hydrogels with a tunable pore size, structure, and degradation rate can be formed with different techniques, including salt leaching, carbon dioxide foaming, and freeze-drying. PLA hydrogel sponges have been used as scaffolds for different cell types in the injured spinal cord, resulting in rather poor cell survival,[8] and a degradable PLA-b-PHEMA block copolymer induces limited axon growth.[9] In a lateral hemisection lesion, PLGA implants, which were copolymerized with polylysine and seeded with an immortalized mouse neural stem cell (NSC) line, have been reported to promote functional recovery in rats.[10] However, the evidence for axonal regeneration underlying this effect is very limited. In a small primate study, similar PLGA sponges seeded with human NSCs were virtually completely degraded after 7 weeks, showing little if any cell survival.[11] A phase I clinical study sponsored by In Vivo Therapeutics (Cambridge, MA) assessing the safety and feasibility of such hydrogels in acute human SCI started in 2014. The primary aim of this study is to demonstrate the safety and feasibility of PLGA implantation into acute sensorimotor complete SCI (http://clinicaltrials.gov/show/ NCT02138110). No adverse effects have been reported to date, indicating a good compatibility of the biomaterial.

Besides hydrogels with a random porous structure, PLA or PLGA scaffolds containing longitudinal oriented micropores, aligned fibers, or channels as guidance matrix for regenerating axons have been examined, such as PLA sponges with longitudinally oriented macropores connected to each other by a network of micropores. Promising in vitro results have shown that aligned PLA microfibers can promote linear neurite growth. To create a 3D scaffold, microfiber sheets can be rolled into conduits, but the large lumen inside the scaffold necessitates a combination with cell seeding or other biomaterials. Microfiber conduits filled with a fibrin gel support higher rostrocaudal axonal growth than do conduits with randomly oriented fibers or a PLA film after complete spinal cord transections.[12]

Macroporous PLA conduits filled with Schwann cells can support the formation of a vascularized tissue bridge containing myelinated axons across the completely transected rat spinal cord. However, the instability of the transplanted scaffolds is detrimental to axonal regeneration.[13] PLGA scaffolds containing a multichannel structure have been used in several studies to promote regeneration. Although they contain a linear channel structure filled with a tissue bridge over a transection lesion, most of these hydrogels are still highly porous and enable cell infiltration and undirected axon regeneration outside of the channels.[14] NSCs and Schwann cells are compatible with the scaffolds and facilitate axonal regeneration into the lesion.[15,16] Irrespective of cell seeding, axonal regeneration across the lesion or functional improvement is not observed. However, in a mouse cervical lateral hemisection model, green fluorescent protein (GFP)-labeled axons in transgenic animals seem to regenerate across a similar PLGA bridge. Whether these axons or this reduced tissue loss/glial scar formation contributes to the small functional recovery remains unclear.[17] Porous multichannel scaffolds have also been used as a matrix for local gene delivery of neurotrophins to increase axon extension into the lesion.[18]

Although aliphatic polyesters have been used extensively in medical applications and have ideal characteristics for the release of therapeutic agents, their utility in soft tissue engineering has limitations due to their stiffness and elastic deformation characteristics, relatively poor survival of seeded cells, fast degradation, and potential loss of structural support.

Hydrogels from Natural Polymers

Natural hydrogel forming polymers based on carbohydrates, glycosaminoglycans, and proteins/peptides have been extensively examined in animal models of SCI. Components of the ECM isolated from mammalian tissue or produced by mammalian cell lines such as collagen and hyaluronic acid, polymers from plants such as agarose and alginate, and chitosan isolated from arthropods belong to this class. Natural polymers are often chemically altered during or after their isolation, and different polymers can be combined into one biomaterial.

Agarose

Agarose is usually extracted from seaweed, dissolves in near-boiling water, and forms a gel after cooling. Other methods to prepare agarose hydrogels are critical point drying and lyophilization to form highly porous hydrogels with different pore diameters, depending on the method and agarose concentration. Gel stiffness can be manipulated by changing the agarose concentration in the sol. Agarose scaffolds are biocompatible and retain their microstructure in the injured spinal cord for at least several weeks.[19]

Agarose hydrogels prepared from hydroxyethylated agarose can be gelled in situ inside the lesion by cooling below 17°C for 30 seconds to fill irregular-shaped spinal cord lesions. The material can serve as a carrier for lipid microtubules releasing neurotrophins,[20] for PLGA nanoparticles for the localized delivery of methylprednisolone, thermostabilized chondroitinase ABC and NT-3, or a combination thereof.[21,22] Overall, these strategies lead to reduced inflammation or enhanced axon growth as expected. However, axons fail to extend throughout the entire lesion or cross into the distal spinal cord.

To provide physical guidance for regenerating axons, agarose hydrogels with a parallel channel structure can be generated by directional freeze-drying or as templated scaffolds with uniform channels. Filling the channel lumen with a collagen matrix containing brain-derived neurotrophic factor (BDNF) significantly enhances the number of regenerating axons inside the channels.[19] Similarly, seeding bone marrow stromal cells (BMSCs) secreting BDNF into the channel enhances the growth of axons (including descending axons) into the scaffold channels.[23] However, axons do not bridge across the lesion site. Even in a model of dorsal column sensory axon injury, combining scaffolds with (1) cells secreting NT-3, (2) activation of the intrinsic growth capacity of sensory axons by a peripheral lesion, and (3) a distal gradient of NT-3 by lentivirus transduction does not enable axon bridging into the spinal parenchyma to make new connections.[24] Thus, an anisotropic channel structure promotes strong linear axon regeneration into the scaffold channels, but a reactive cell matrix forming at the interface of the implant and the spinal parenchyma limits regeneration beyond the lesion site. This problem is not unique to agarose scaffolds, but rather is an overall obstacle encountered with all biomaterials that aim to promote axon bridging across the lesion site.

Alginate

Alginate is a heteromeric polysaccharide isolated from several brown algae species.[25] Alginate salts with monovalent cations like sodium (Na^+) are soluble in water. By exchange of these cations with multivalent cations (e.g., Ca^{2+} or Sr^{2+}), hydrogels are formed by ionotropic cross-linking. A similar effect can be obtained by chemical cross-linking of the polysaccharide chains. The stiffness of the gel depends on the overall molecular weight and concentration of alginate and the distribution of the different monomer blocks. Guluronic acid-rich alginate forms stronger and more ductile hydrogels by ionotropic cross-linking compared with mannuronic acid-rich alginates. The type of cross-linking agent and the cross-linking density also influence the mechanical properties of the hydrogel. Due to the carboxylic acid groups, alginate is negatively charged under physiological conditions, which adversely affects cells and leads to a reduced neurite outgrowth. However, alginate hydrogels can be coated with positively charged molecules such as poly-L-ornithine or chemically modified to mask their negative surface charge.[26] Alginate is basically not biodegradable, but ionically (not chemically) cross-linked alginate hydrogels dissolve into single polymer strands by exchanging the cross-linking multivalent cations for monovalent cations.

In several experiments, alginate hydrogels have been used to encapsulate BDNF-secreting fibroblasts to isolate cells from the host immune system and thereby enhance their survival. The continued secretion of BDNF can promote axonal regeneration in the surrounding host parenchyma and some functional recovery.[27] Injectable alginate hydrogels have also been used as a matrix for the sustained release of growth factors in combination with PLGA-based microparticles or chitosan-dextran sulfate nanoparticles to promote neurite growth or infiltration of endothelial cells. A downside of injectable alginate hydrogels is the high concentration of divalent cations like calcium needed to gel the alginate solution, which can have cytotoxic effects.

Alginate scaffolds with a channel structure produced by directed diffusion of divalent cations and subsequent stabilization with an interpenetrating polyurea network formed by the polymerization of hexamethylene diisocyanate can promote linear axonal regeneration in rat spinal cord transections. In an entorhinal-hippocampal slice culture model as well as in a dorsal column lesion in adult rats, alginate scaffolds with capillaries of 27-µm diameter promote longitudinally oriented axonal regeneration.[28] Similar to studies with agarose-based hydrogel channels, alginates with channel structure can guide axons parallel to the channel walls in rostrocaudal direction. In combination with BMSCs expressing BDNF, axons extend over longer distances within the channels compared with lesions that are filled only with cells, where axons have a random growth orientation.[29] As described above, axon bridging into the distal spinal cord is not observed, and chemically stabilized alginate scaffolds are not biodegradable after 6 weeks in vivo.

Results of these experiments suggest that alginate hydrogels can provide a permissive microenvironment for regeneration of spinal cord axons. The beneficial effect of alginate scaffolds can be enhanced by masking the negative charge of the hydrogel by protein coating. In combination with cell seeding and growth factor release, and by using hydrogels with parallel channel structure, oriented axonal regeneration can be further enhanced. However, the formation of a reactive cell layer around the hydrogels is one hurdle that remains to be overcome.

Chitosan

Chitosan, a linear polysaccharide produced by deacetylation of chitin from the exoskeleton of crustaceans and insects, is water soluble depending on the degree of deacetylation.[30] Chitosan and its degradation products have displayed neuroprotective and antioxidative activity.[30] The mechanical properties of chitosan-based hydrogels can be altered by chemical cross-linking or incorporation of a second polymer network penetrating the chitosan matrix.

Chitosan hydrogels with a channel structure have been used as a scaffold in the injured spinal cord to guide the growth of axons. They do not elicit a chronic immune response and remain stable in the spinal cord for at least 12 months.[31] Chitosan channels with peripheral nerve grafts implanted 1 or 4 weeks after a compression injury contain a tissue bridge with a large amount of myelinated axons after 14 weeks in vivo.[32] Similarly, neural progenitor cells (NPCs) seeded in laminin-coated scaffolds survive, differentiate into glia, and host axons and blood vessels extend into the scaffold.[33] Several combinatory strategies using chitosan channels have been examined to enhance the survival of NPCs, including dibutyryl cyclic adenosine monophosphate (cAMP) encapsulated within PLGA microspheres.[34] Despite providing a tissue bridge across the lesion site, growth of axons beyond the scaffolds or recovery of locomotor function was not observed. Although stable chitosan scaffolds provide long-lasting structural support, the missing biodegradability also raises some concern. Taken together, only combined with (stem) cell or peripheral nerve grafts, chitosan hydrogels are able to provide a scaffold for the formation of a tissue bridge over a lesion site.

Collagen

Collagen is one of the most abundant proteins in mammals and an important structural ECM protein supporting cells with a physical scaffold and biochemical cues. The protein mainly occurs as triple helix fibrils (type 1 collagen) that can form a self-assembling hydrogel, which is biodegradable and therefore frequently cross-linked to stabilize its structure and physical properties. The stiffness of the scaffold and its degradation rate depend on the chemical properties and concentration of the molecules used for cross-linking. Collagen is one of the best-characterized biomaterials in medical applications. Collagen matrices have been used as scaffolds and vehicles for the transplantation of various cell types and for growth factor release enhancing the survival of Schwann cells and increasing the number of axons growing into the scaffold.[35]

Collagen-based biomaterials have also been used to graft fibroblasts genetically modified to express neurotrophic factors (reviewed in

McCall et al[36]). Although some studies transplanted cross-linked collagen scaffolds in combination with different axon growth-promoting strategies (Nogo receptor, chondroitinase ABC [ChABC], stem cells) to the spinal cord, the amount of axon sprouting into the lesion is rather limited. Collagen scaffolds composed of aligned collagen filaments might be an interesting alternative to promote rostrocaudally oriented axonal regeneration.[37] Incorporation of BDNF with a collagen binding domain into a scaffold of aligned collagen fibers increases axon growth, and supposedly some functional recovery after a complete transection in a canine model.[38] Other means to obtain directional axon growth might be collagen hydrogels with a honeycomb[39] or channel structure,[40] or conduits with larger channels and aligned fibers.[41] Although these approaches in combination with BMSC or plasmid-based NT-3 delivery increase axon sprouting or enhance some recovery of forepaw function compared with lesion-only controls, axons do not regenerate across the scaffold, and the orientation of axons has not been examined.

Fibrin

Fibrin, an important factor in blood coagulation, is generated by thrombin-mediated cleavage of soluble fibrinogen into fibrin monomers, which spontaneously form fibers that give rise to a fibrin hydrogel. This enzymatic reaction can be used for a biological two-component glue, and the fast biodegradability can be reduced by inclusion of protease inhibitors.[42]

Fibrin hydrogels grafted to a spinal cord lesion induces some neurite sprouting and seems to reduce astrogliosis around the lesion site.[43] In combination with fibronectin, axon sprouting into the hydrogel slightly increases.[44] There are some hints that salmon fibrin instead of mammalian fibrin has the potential for higher axonal sparing.[45] In combination with the knockdown of PTEN (phosphatase and tensin homologue deleted on chromosome 10) in the cortex to improve the neuron-intrinsic growth capacity, the injection of salmon fibrin into a dorsal hemisection enhances growth of corticospinal axons and to some extent the

recovery of voluntary motor function.[46] Fibrin hydrogels placed epidurally on a lesion have also been used for the delivery of chondroitinase ABC, reducing the level of inhibitory chondroitin sulfate proteoglycans (CSPGs) more than a single intraparenchymal injection.[47]

Fibrin glues have also been used as a substrate for cell transplantation. Mixing cells suspended in a solution of fibrinogen and thrombin to form a gel enhances cell survival. NSCs embedded into such a matrix with a growth factor cocktail have shown excellent survival and extensive long-distance axonal outgrowth after grafting to a full transection site.[48] The fast degradability of fibrin is not ideal for a sustained release of therapeutic agents. Therefore, a chemically modified fibrin has been developed, with immobilized heparin to temporarily bind heparin-binding growth factors. The release of neurotrophins from such modified hydrogels leads to a minor, dose-dependent increase in axon sprouting.[49] In addition, the survival and proliferation of NPCs and embryonic stem (ES) cell–derived progenitor motor neurons is enhanced in a fibrin matrix releasing NT-3 and platelet-derived growth factor (PDGF).[50–52]

Fibrin glues have been extensively utilized in studies transplanting peripheral nerve grafts. Based on preclinical results that showed a functional improvement after acidic FGF-1 administration from fibrin glue in the completely transected rat spinal cord that received peripheral nerve implants,[53] a phase I clinical trial was initiated. A fibrin glue containing FGF-1 was implanted in chronic SCI patients after laminectomy, and an adjuvant booster of combined FGF-1 and fibrin glue was given intrathecally at 3 and 6 months postsurgery. Although the feasibility and safety of this administration technique has been established, the efficacy of the therapy remains to be determined.[54]

Thus, fibrin hydrogels have been shown to be highly biocompatible and biodegradable. Although fibrin is not able to support substantial axonal regeneration on its own, in combination with sustained growth factor release and cell therapy, it can be a useful tool to promote tissue regeneration.

Hyaluronic Acid

The glycosaminoglycan hyaluronic acid is a main structural component of the ECM in the CNS. Hyaluronic acid is a linear disaccharide polymer that can absorb large amounts of water. A reduction of its high water solubility and fast biodegradation, and an adjustment of its stiffness, is possible by esterification of the carboxylic acid groups of the D-glucuronic acid subunit,[55] cross-linking of the hyaluronic acid chains,[56] or combination with other materials such as methylcellulose.[57] In terms of axonal regeneration, there is no evidence that chemically cross-linked hyaluronic acid hydrogels implanted into the injured spinal cord can provide, independent of their degradability, a structural scaffold for axon regeneration. However, hyaluronic acid and especially the blend of hyaluronic acid and methylcellulose have some potential for reducing scarring and subarachnoid inflammation, leading to a modest increase in locomotor function,[57] or as a matrix for the sustained release of therapeutic agents such as growth factors.[58] In vitro and in vivo experiments have also shown the potential of injectable hyaluronic acid–methylcellulose hydrogels as a cell delivery system. NPCs incorporated into a hydrogel blend can reduce cavitation and promote higher neuronal sparing compared with cell injection without the hydrogel matrix.[59] Several different covalently cross-linked hyaluronic acid hydrogels have been produced to enhance the mechanical characteristics but do not seem to permit axonal growth. However, injected into the intrathecal space, covalently cross-linked hydrogels are biocompatible and a potential matrix for the release of growth factors.[60]

Matrigel

Matrigel™ (Corning Life Sciences, Durham, NC) is a soluble extract of basement membrane proteins from a mouse sarcoma cell line. It is a poorly defined mixture of more than 1,800 proteins including ECM components and a variety of growth factors and proteins related to the binding and signaling of growth factors.[61] This is a major shortcoming, as the exact composition varies between batches, making it more difficult to replicate findings and limiting clinical applications. As Matrigel is soluble at 4°C and forms a 3D gel at 37°C, it is ideal for covering the surface of cell culture plastic ware and for injecting into spinal cord lesion cavities. Matrigel alone has only limited potential to promote axonal regeneration in the injured spinal cord, but it has proven its utility as a matrix for cell transplantation, enhancing the survival of transplanted cells. Studies with Schwann cells also indicate that in vivo gelation is superior to the implantation of pre-gelled Matrigel.[62] Matrigel has been used to fill the lumen of a semipermeable polyacrylonitrile/polyvinylchloride (PAN/PVC) copolymer channels, and, in combination with Schwann cells, unmyelinated and myelinated axons and blood vessels extend into the grafts. There is also some evidence suggesting that axons are able to grow across the graft and reenter the intact host tissue when growth factors are provided in the distal host spinal cord.[36]

Self-Assembling Peptides

Peptide amphiphiles (PAs) represent a class of peptide-based biomolecules that spontaneously self-assemble into well-defined nanostructures such as fibrils, nanofibers, and spherical micelles or vesicles. In physiological media or aqueous solution, self-assembly is driven by an intermolecular interplay of ionic or hydrophobic interactions between complementary amphiphilic peptide structures under certain conditions (e.g., pH, temperature, ionic strength).[63] For tissue engineering and biomedical applications, bioactive peptide epitopes can be incorporated into self-assembling peptides (SAPs) to be displayed on the surface affecting cell survival, cellular behavior, and differentiation.[64,65] Embedding cells in SAPs has shown some promise in restoring function after SCI; PA displaying the laminin epitope IKVAV promoted axon regeneration, suppressed glial scar formation, increased oligodendroglial differentiation, and partially restored motor function.[66] Recently, a combination of bioactive SAPs and NSCs also improved forelimb motor recovery by decreasing cystic cavitation and motor neurons death after cervical SCI.[67]

Conclusion

A large variety of biomaterials derived from natural and synthetic polymers have been investigated for their efficacy in spinal cord regeneration. Although fully synthetic materials have well-defined chemical and physical properties, they often have to be modified to better match the biological characteristics of the spinal cord. More studies have investigated materials derived from natural polymers in the injured spinal cord. Independent of their origin, hydrogels can serve as scaffolds to provide structural or directional support in a lesion site, as matrices for transplanted cells, and as vehicles for the release of growth factors, gene vectors, and other therapeutic agents, with the goal of promoting axon regeneration and replacing tissue lost after SCI. Several studies using biomaterials have reported functional recovery, but many of these studies are difficult to interpret, lack thorough data, and therefore fail to convincingly describe any mechanism underlying the observed behavioral effect. Indeed, no conclusive publication has clearly demonstrated functional improvement using biomaterials without any additional combinatory treatment. Of the publications combining biomaterials with other treatments, recovery is often minimal, only a very small number of animals are investigated, or histological data are not interpretable and do not provide a proper explanation for the observed effects. Therefore, it is not surprising that only a few materials have moved toward larger animals models or clinical studies despite huge advancements in the field. However, it is conceivable that more detailed studies in lesion models that better reproduce neuropathological mechanisms of human injuries, such as spinal cord contusions or compressions, will be initiated in the near future as knowledge about biomaterials and the combination with other treatments is rapidly increasing.

Chapter Summary

Considerable progress has been made in the last decade in the development of biomaterials suitable for grafting to the injured spinal cord. Hydrogel-based materials are particularly versatile as many biochemical and physical properties can be adjusted to match the stiffness and elasticity of the spinal cord, and surfaces can be modified for better biocompatibility. Natural and/or synthetic polymers such as self-assembling peptides can support survival of graft- and host-derived cells. Materials with anisotropic structures such as alginates and agarose can promote directed axon regeneration, and several biomaterials have shown promise for localized drug delivery. Thus, hydrogels can serve as a platform for parallel, combinatory treatment approaches that are likely required for significant functional improvements, particularly after severe SCI. This chapter summarized recent advances in hydrogel polymers in combination with cell and drug delivery in the injured spinal cord and discussed some of the current challenges.

Pearls

- ◆ A wide variety of biomaterials with very good biocompatibility are now available.
- ◆ The physical guidance of axons through hydrogel channels is possible.
- ◆ Combinatorial approaches of cellular therapies with biomaterials in many cases are superior to cell therapy alone.
- ◆ Substantial progress is being made in chemical and biochemical modifications of hydrogels for cell and drug delivery in the injured spinal cord.

Pitfalls

- ◆ Numerous claims for functional recovery in animal models are made without an understanding of the mechanisms.
- ◆ Biomaterials alone seem insufficient for axon regeneration across a lesion in the spinal cord.
- ◆ There has been only limited clinical translation of biomaterials in SCI.

References

Five Must-Read References

1. Gu X, Ding F, Yang Y, Liu J. Construction of tissue engineered nerve grafts and their application in peripheral nerve regeneration. Prog Neurobiol 2011; 93:204–230

2. Estrada V, Brazda N, Schmitz C, et al. Long-lasting significant functional improvement in chronic severe spinal cord injury following scar resection and polyethylene glycol implantation. Neurobiol Dis 2014; 67:165–179

3. Hakim JS, Esmaeili Rad M, Grahn PJ, et al. Positively charged oligo[poly(ethylene glycol) fumarate] scaffold implantation results in a permissive lesion environment after spinal cord injury in rat. Tissue Eng Part A 2015;21:2099–2114

4. Piantino J, Burdick JA, Goldberg D, Langer R, Benowitz LI. An injectable, biodegradable hydrogel for trophic factor delivery enhances axonal rewiring and improves performance after spinal cord injury. Exp Neurol 2006;201:359–367

5. Chen B, He J, Yang H, et al. Repair of spinal cord injury by implantation of bFGF-incorporated HEMA-MOETACL hydrogel in rats. Sci Rep 2015;5:9017

6. Tsai EC, Dalton PD, Shoichet MS, Tator CH. Matrix inclusion within synthetic hydrogel guidance channels improves specific supraspinal and local axonal regeneration after complete spinal cord transection. Biomaterials 2006;27:519–533

7. Woerly S, Doan VD, Sosa N, de Vellis J, Espinosa A. Reconstruction of the transected cat spinal cord following NeuroGel implantation: axonal tracing, immunohistochemical and ultrastructural studies. Int J Dev Neurosci 2001;19:63–83

8. Deumens R, Koopmans GC, Honig WM, et al. Olfactory ensheathing cells, olfactory nerve fibroblasts and biomatrices to promote long-distance axon regrowth and functional recovery in the dorsally hemisected adult rat spinal cord. Exp Neurol 2006;200:89–103

9. Pertici V, Trimaille T, Laurin J, et al. Repair of the injured spinal cord by implantation of a synthetic degradable block copolymer in rat. Biomaterials 2014;35:6248–6258

10. Teng YD, Lavik EB, Qu X, et al. Functional recovery following traumatic spinal cord injury mediated by a unique polymer scaffold seeded with neural stem cells. Proc Natl Acad Sci U S A 2002;99:3024–3029

11. Pritchard CD, Slotkin JR, Yu D, et al. Establishing a model spinal cord injury in the African green monkey for the preclinical evaluation of biodegradable polymer scaffolds seeded with human neural stem cells. J Neurosci Methods 2010;188:258–269

12. Hurtado A, Cregg JM, Wang HB, et al. Robust CNS regeneration after complete spinal cord transection using aligned poly-L-lactic acid microfibers. Biomaterials 2011;32:6068–6079

13. Oudega M, Gautier SE, Chapon P, et al. Axonal regeneration into Schwann cell grafts within resorbable poly(alpha-hydroxyacid) guidance channels in the adult rat spinal cord. Biomaterials 2001;22:1125–1136

14. Yang Y, De Laporte L, Zelivyanskaya ML, et al. Multiple channel bridges for spinal cord injury: cellular characterization of host response. Tissue Eng Part A 2009;15:3283–3295

15. Olson HE, Rooney GE, Gross L, et al. Neural stem cell- and Schwann cell-loaded biodegradable polymer scaffolds support axonal regeneration in the transected spinal cord. Tissue Eng Part A 2009;15:1797–1805

16. Chen BK, Knight AM, de Ruiter GCW, et al. Axon regeneration through scaffold into distal spinal cord after transection. J Neurotrauma 2009;26:1759–1771

17. Pawar K, Cummings BJ, Thomas A, et al. Biomaterial bridges enable regeneration and re-entry of corticospinal tract axons into the caudal spinal cord after SCI: Association with recovery of forelimb function. Biomaterials 2015;65:1–12

18. Tuinstra HM, Aviles MO, Shin S, et al. Multifunctional, multichannel bridges that deliver neurotrophin encoding lentivirus for regeneration following spinal cord injury. Biomaterials 2012;33:1618–1626

19. Stokols S, Tuszynski MH. Freeze-dried agarose scaffolds with uniaxial channels stimulate and guide linear axonal growth following spinal cord injury. Biomaterials 2006;27:443–451

20. Jain A, Kim YT, McKeon RJ, Bellamkonda RV. In situ gelling hydrogels for conformal repair of spinal cord defects, and local delivery of BDNF after spinal cord injury. Biomaterials 2006;27:497–504

21. Lee H, McKeon RJ, Bellamkonda RV. Sustained delivery of thermostabilized chABC enhances axonal sprouting and functional recovery after spinal cord injury. Proc Natl Acad Sci U S A 2010;107:3340–3345

22. Chvatal SA, Kim YT, Bratt-Leal AM, Lee H, Bellamkonda RV. Spatial distribution and acute anti-inflammatory effects of methylprednisolone after sustained local delivery to the contused spinal cord. Biomaterials 2008;29:1967–1975

23. Gao M, Lu P, Bednark B, et al. Templated agarose scaffolds for the support of motor axon regeneration into sites of complete spinal cord transection. Biomaterials 2013;34:1529–1536

24. Gros T, Sakamoto JS, Blesch A, Havton LA, Tuszynski MH. Regeneration of long-tract axons through sites of spinal cord injury using templated agarose scaffolds. Biomaterials 2010;31:6719–6729

25. Augst AD, Kong HJ, Mooney DJ. Alginate hydrogels as biomaterials. Macromol Biosci 2006;6:623–633

26. Tobias CA, Dhoot NO, Wheatley MA, Tessler A, Murray M, Fischer I. Grafting of encapsulated BDNF-producing fibroblasts into the injured spinal cord without immune suppression in adult rats. J Neurotrauma 2001;18:287–301

27. Tobias CA, Han SS, Shumsky JS, et al. Alginate encapsulated BDNF-producing fibroblast grafts permit recovery of function after spinal cord injury in the absence of immune suppression. J Neurotrauma 2005;22: 138–156

28. Prang P, Müller R, Eljaouhari A, et al. The promotion of oriented axonal regrowth in the injured spinal cord by alginate-based anisotropic capillary hydrogels. Biomaterials 2006;27:3560–3569

29. Günther MI, Weidner N, Müller R, Blesch A. Cell-seeded alginate hydrogel scaffolds promote directed linear axonal regeneration in the injured rat spinal cord. Acta Biomater 2015;27:140–150

30. Zou P, Yang X, Wang J, et al. Advances in characterisation and biological activities of chitosan and chitosan oligosaccharides. Food Chem 2016;190:1174–1181

31. Kim H, Tator CH, Shoichet MS. Chitosan implants in the rat spinal cord: biocompatibility and biodegradation. J Biomed Mater Res A 2011;97:395–404

32. Nomura H, Baladie B, Katayama Y, Morshead CM, Shoichet MS, Tator CH. Delayed implantation of intramedullary chitosan channels containing nerve grafts promotes extensive axonal regeneration after spinal cord injury. Neurosurgery 2008;63:127–141, discussion 141–143

33. Nomura H, Zahir T, Kim H, et al. Extramedullary chitosan channels promote survival of transplanted neural stem and progenitor cells and create a tissue bridge after complete spinal cord transection. Tissue Eng Part A 2008;14:649–665

34. Kim H, Zahir T, Tator CH, Shoichet MS. Effects of dibutyryl cyclic-AMP on survival and neuronal differentiation of neural stem/progenitor cells transplanted into spinal cord injured rats. PLoS ONE 2011;6:e21744

35. Patel V, Joseph G, Patel A, et al. Suspension matrices for improved Schwann-cell survival after implantation into the injured rat spinal cord. J Neurotrauma 2010;27:789–801

36. McCall J, Weidner N, Blesch A. Neurotrophic factors in combinatorial approaches for spinal cord regeneration. Cell Tissue Res 2012;349:27–37

37. Liu T, Houle JD, Xu J, Chan BP, Chew SY. Nanofibrous collagen nerve conduits for spinal cord repair. Tissue Eng Part A 2012;18:1057–1066

38. Han S, Wang B, Jin W, et al. The linear-ordered collagen scaffold-BDNF complex significantly promotes functional recovery after completely transected spinal cord injury in canine. Biomaterials 2015;41:89–96

39. Onuma-Ukegawa M, Bhatt K, Hirai T, et al. Bone marrow stromal cells combined with a honeycomb collagen sponge facilitate neurite elongation in vitro and neural restoration in the hemisected rat spinal cord. Cell Transplant 2015;24:1283–1297

40. Altinova H, Möllers S, Führmann T, et al. Functional improvement following implantation of a microstructured, type-I collagen scaffold into experimental injuries of the adult rat spinal cord. Brain Res 2014;1585:37–50

41. Yao L, Daly W, Newland B, et al. Improved axonal regeneration of transected spinal cord mediated by multichannel collagen conduits functionalized with neurotrophin-3 gene. Gene Ther 2013;20:1149–1157

42. Lorentz KM, Kontos S, Frey P, Hubbell JA. Engineered aprotinin for improved stability of fibrin biomaterials. Biomaterials 2011;32:430–438

43. Johnson PJ, Parker SR, Sakiyama-Elbert SE. Fibrin-based tissue engineering scaffolds enhance neural fiber sprouting and delay the accumulation of reactive astrocytes at the lesion in a subacute model of spinal cord injury. J Biomed Mater Res A 2010;92: 152–163

44. King VR, Alovskaya A, Wei DY, Brown RA, Priestley JV. The use of injectable forms of fibrin and fibronectin to support axonal ingrowth after spinal cord injury. Biomaterials 2010;31:4447–4456

45. Sharp KG, Dickson AR, Marchenko SA, et al. Salmon fibrin treatment of spinal cord injury promotes functional recovery and density of serotonergic innervation. Exp Neurol 2012;235:345–356

46. Lewandowski G, Steward O. AAVshRNA-mediated suppression of PTEN in adult rats in combination with salmon fibrin administration enables regenerative growth of corticospinal axons and enhances recovery of voluntary motor function after cervical spinal cord injury. J Neurosci 2014;34:9951–9962

47. Hyatt AJ, Wang D, Kwok JC, Fawcett JW, Martin KR. Controlled release of chondroitinase ABC from fibrin gel reduces the level of inhibitory glycosaminoglycan chains in lesioned spinal cord. J Control Release 2010;147:24–29

48. Lu P, Wang Y, Graham L, et al. Long-distance growth and connectivity of neural stem cells after severe spinal cord injury. Cell 2012;150:1264–1273

49. Taylor SJ, Rosenzweig ES, McDonald JW III, Sakiyama-Elbert SE. Delivery of neurotrophin-3 from fibrin enhances neuronal fiber sprouting after spinal cord injury. J Control Release 2006;113:226–235

50. Johnson PJ, Tatara A, McCreedy DA, Shiu A, Sakiyama-Elbert SE. Tissue-engineered fibrin scaffolds containing neural progenitors enhance functional recovery in a subacute model of SCI. Soft Matter 2010;6:5127–5137

51. Johnson PJ, Tatara A, Shiu A, Sakiyama-Elbert SE. Controlled release of neurotrophin-3 and platelet-derived growth factor from fibrin scaffolds containing neural progenitor cells enhances survival and

differentiation into neurons in a subacute model of SCI. Cell Transplant 2010;19:89–101

52. McCreedy DA, Wilems TS, Xu H, et al. Survival, differentiation, and migration of high-purity mouse embryonic stem cell-derived progenitor motor neurons in fibrin scaffolds after sub-acute spinal cord injury. Biomater Sci 2014;2:1672–1682

53. Cheng H, Cao Y, Olson L. Spinal cord repair in adult paraplegic rats: partial restoration of hind limb function. Science 1996;273:510–513

54. Wu JC, Huang WC, Chen YC, et al. Acidic fibroblast growth factor for repair of human spinal cord injury: a clinical trial. J Neurosurg Spine 2011;15:216–227

55. Campoccia D, Doherty P, Radice M, Brun P, Abatangelo G, Williams DF. Semisynthetic resorbable materials from hyaluronan esterification. Biomaterials 1998;19:2101–2127

56. Bencherif SA, Srinivasan A, Horkay F, Hollinger JO, Matyjaszewski K, Washburn NR. Influence of the degree of methacrylation on hyaluronic acid hydrogels properties. Biomaterials 2008;29:1739–1749

57. Austin JW, Kang CE, Baumann MD, et al. The effects of intrathecal injection of a hyaluronan-based hydrogel on inflammation, scarring and neurobehavioural outcomes in a rat model of severe spinal cord injury associated with arachnoiditis. Biomaterials 2012;33:4555–4564

58. Gupta D, Tator CH, Shoichet MS. Fast-gelling injectable blend of hyaluronan and methylcellulose for intrathecal, localized delivery to the injured spinal cord. Biomaterials 2006;27:2370–2379

59. Mothe AJ, Tam RY, Zahir T, Tator CH, Shoichet MS. Repair of the injured spinal cord by transplantation of neural stem cells in a hyaluronan-based hydrogel. Biomaterials 2013;34:3775–3783

60. Führmann T, Obermeyer J, Tator CH, Shoichet MS. Click-crosslinked injectable hyaluronic acid hydrogel is safe and biocompatible in the intrathecal space for ultimate use in regenerative strategies of the injured spinal cord. Methods 2015;84:60–69

61. Hughes CS, Postovit LM, Lajoie GA. Matrigel: a complex protein mixture required for optimal growth of cell culture. Proteomics 2010;10:1886–1890

62. Williams RR, Henao M, Pearse DD, Bunge MB. Permissive Schwann cell graft/spinal cord interfaces for axon regeneration. Cell Transplant 2015;24:115–131

63. Dehsorkhi A, Castelletto V, Hamley IW. Self-assembling amphiphilic peptides. J Pept Sci 2014;20:453–467

64. Silva GA, Czeisler C, Niece KL, et al. Selective differentiation of neural progenitor cells by high-epitope density nanofibers. Science 2004;303:1352–1355

65. Webber MJ, Tongers J, Renault MA, Roncalli JG, Losordo DW, Stupp SI. Development of bioactive peptide amphiphiles for therapeutic cell delivery. Acta Biomater 2010;6:3–11

66. Tysseling-Mattiace VM, Sahni V, Niece KL, et al. Self-assembling nanofibers inhibit glial scar formation and promote axon elongation after spinal cord injury. J Neurosci 2008;28:3814–3823

67. Iwasaki M, Wilcox JT, Nishimura Y, et al. Synergistic effects of self-assembling peptide and neural stem/progenitor cells to promote tissue repair and forelimb functional recovery in cervical spinal cord injury. Biomaterials 2014;35:2617–2629

10

Neural Stem Cell Transplantation for Spinal Cord Repair

Ina K. Simeonova, Beatrice Sandner, and Norbert Weidner

■ Introduction

Every few months, breaking news of innovative therapies suggest another imminent cure for a variety of neurologic disorders, including spinal cord injury (SCI). Careful analyses of the reported findings indicate that proof-of-principle results have been achieved. Unfortunately, these results are by no means sufficient to expect a clinically relevant therapeutic approach in the near future. Nevertheless, in recent years significant progress has been made, which helped dramatically to move the field forward step by step toward a clinical application. This chapter summarizes the current status of neural stem cell (NSC)-based transplantation strategies on the preclinical and clinical level.

Traumatic injury to the spine with consecutive compression/contusion of the spinal cord and cauda equina represents the most common cause of spinal cord disease. As a result, long descending and ascending axon pathways traversing the injury site get transected or demyelinated, and neurons at the level of injury undergo cell death. Depending on the injury level and severity, profound sensorimotor (para/tetraparesis) and autonomous dysfunction (bladder, bowel, sexual, cardiovascular, respiratory dysfunction) is the consequence.

In contrast to the peripheral nervous system, transected axons in the central nervous system (CNS) do not spontaneously regenerate,

and degenerated neurons will not be replaced (**Fig. 10.1a**). Remyelination occurs only to a limited degree. Furthermore, key factors such as degeneration of injured spinal cord tissue with consecutive fibroglial scar and cystic cavity formation, upregulation of growth inhibitory factors, and a lack of sufficient intrinsic axon regrowth capacity prevent intrinsic tissue repair.[1]

In incomplete SCI, functional recovery can be achieved by neurorehabilitative interventions aiming for restoration of body functions. Their success depends on the degree of incompleteness. In patients with complete SCI, the lost sensorimotor and autonomous function cannot be restored. Specialized SCI centers can provide comprehensive rehabilitative care, which enables respective patients to gain independence by means of compensatory strategies (e.g., wheelchair mobility to substitute for lost walking function, intermittent self-catheterization to empty the bladder). In these cases only powerful regenerative therapies will be able to recreate the structural basis for functional recovery. Cystic lesion defects need to be bridged with appropriate substrates to enable axon regrowth across the lesion site, inhibitory molecules need to be blocked, the intrinsic axonal growth capacity needs to be enhanced, and regenerating axons need to be (re)myelinated.[2]

It is widely agreed that these different mechanisms need to be addressed in combination

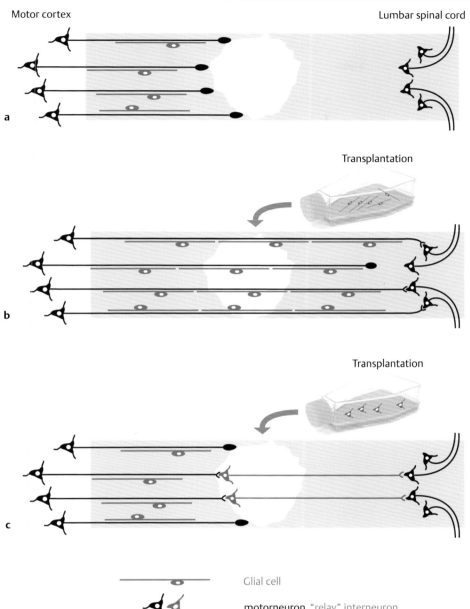

Motor cortex

Lumbar spinal cord

a

Transplantation

b

Transplantation

c

——————●—————— Glial cell

◄◄ motorneuron, "relay" interneuron

Fig. 10.1 Traumatic lesion of the spinal cord *(gray)* exemplified by the descending motor pathways (corticospinal tract). **(a)** Descending axons derived from the upper motoneurons located in the motor cortex become transected by the traumatic spinal cord lesion (cystic lesion defect shown in *white*), which interrupts the connectivity to the lower motoneurons located caudal to the injury site with the functional consequence of para- or tetraparesis depending on the level of injury. **(b)** Suitable neural stem/progenitor cells, for example astroglial cells *(green)*, can help to bridge the cystic lesion defect. Transected motor axon start to regrow across the lesion, and ideally reconnect to previous target neurons with consecutive functional recovery. **(c)** Alternatively, regrowing descending axons connect to neuronally differentiated stem cell grafts, which act as relays and send projections down the caudal spinal cord connecting to lower motoneurons.

to achieve relevant structural and functional recovery after SCI. A combinatorial strategy, which includes factors neutralizing inhibitory factors, promoting axon growth intrinsic capacity, and scaffolds/cells replacing the lost spinal cord tissue, might be feasible in principle. However, considering just the regulatory aspects on the way toward a clinical translation, such combinatorial approaches will become difficult to implement. Ideally, a combinatorial treatment can be integrated into stem cell transplantation alone without having to administer multiple factors, cells, or substrates.

Rationales for Neural Stem Cell–Based Therapies

A stem cell–based therapy following SCI needs to address the following aspects: stem cells need to remyelinate axons in the injured spinal cord; and either spared axons need to be remyelinated or regenerating axons need to be myelinated to restore proper nerve conduction. Recent and ongoing stem cell transplantation strategies, employing embryonic or fetal spinal cord–derived NSC, target this mechanism[3] and have been applied in a phase I/II clinical trial that was first performed by Geron Corp. (Menlo Park, CA) and thereafter taken over by Asterias Biotherapeutics (Fremont, CA).[4] However, a strategy solely focusing on remyelination of spared axons is unlikely to yield substantial functional recovery. The most obvious means to restore function is by enhancing long-distance regeneration (**Fig. 10.1b**). However, this strategy is also the most difficult one. A typically cystic (fluid-filled) lesion defect has to be filled by an appropriate cellular bridge, which facilitates axon regrowth across the lesion defect and directs these regrowing axons toward their previous target neurons. In the end, these axons have to be myelinated appropriately. As mentioned above, just providing a cellular bridge for axon regrowth will most likely not be sufficient to elicit substantial axon regeneration. Extracellular matrix– and myelin-associated axon growth inhibitory molecules need to be blocked, and the intrinsic neuronal

regrowth capacity needs to be enhanced. Another concept remains to be proven in respect to its functionality. As a prerequisite, neural stem or progenitor cells transplanted into the injury site should become neurons. Subsequently, host axons need to regenerate toward and connect to graft-derived neurons, which grow into the host spinal cord and reconnect to denervated target neurons, thus acting as "relay" neurons (**Fig. 10.1c**). Studies investigating both stem cell grafting and spontaneous recovery in incomplete SCI propose such a relay mechanism to yield recovery of locomotor function.[5–7] However, whether such a relay mechanism is really functionally relevant has yet to be determined.

Mechanisms Underlying Neural Stem Cell–Based Therapeutic Effects

Thus far, there is very limited evidence clearly and unequivocally demonstrating axon regeneration over longer distances, with target reinnervation or remyelination of demyelinated axons leading to functional improvement. Proof-of-principle studies have shown that ascending sensory axons can regrow through a growth factor overexpressing stem cell graft back into the host cord and reinnervate target neurons in the brainstem.[8] In respect to long descending motor pathways such as the corticospinal tract, some regrowth supported by glial differentiated neural stem/progenitor cells can be achieved, but substantial long-distance regrowth with reconnection of target neurons has yet to be demonstrated.[9–11]

Robustness of Therapeutic Effects

Besides confirming a relevant structural mechanism for functional repair, another challenge is to induce a robust regenerative response in the injured adult mammalian CNS. A recent study demonstrated for the first time that massive axon outgrowth across long distances can be achieved in the completely transected adult rat spinal cord after grafting E14 rat spinal cord or fetal human spinal cord–derived stem cells in combination with a growth factor cocktail and a fibrinogen/thrombin matrix for better graft survival.[5] As mentioned above, in this study a relay mechanism has been proposed to account for the observed improved hind-limb motor function evaluated according to the Basso, Beattie, and Bresnahan (BBB) open field locomotor rating scale.

The Neuronal Relay Concept

The classic structural repair mechanism in the injured spinal cord requires that transected long descending motor or ascending sensory pathways regrow all the way across the lesion site back into the adjacent host spinal cord and beyond to reinnervate their previous target neurons. Currently, very few studies can dem-onstrate substantial regrowth of injured axons into, and for long distances beyond, the injury site. In some cases, few axons have been identi-fied to reenter the intact spinal cord but only for a very short distance. An alternative strategy— neuronal "relay" formation—uses grafts capa-ble of generating neurons within the injury site to function as interneurons between the tran-sected axons and target neurons. In this sce-nario, transected axons do not need to regrow for long distances, whereas graft-derived neu-rons can be selected/manipulated to promote long-distance axonal outgrowth. Such a relay mechanism has been demonstrated in the con-text of spontaneous structural rearrangement along the corticospinal tract.[7] Task-specific training is most likely required in order to functionally integrate such relays into the cir-cuit.[6] Proof of concept for a functional relay has been shown in a C1 dorsal column transection model, where host sensory axons formed syn-apses with neurons from rat E14.5 neuronal pre-cursor cell grafts.[12] Grafted neuron-restricted precursor cells differentiated and formed syn-apses in nearby dorsal column nuclei in the

caudal brainstem. Electrophysiological record-ings confirmed the functional relevance of this newly formed network. As mentioned, a revis-ited NSC grafting approach—dissociated E14 rat spinal cord in combination with a variety of growth factors—resulted in robust axonal out-growth of graft-derived neurons, synapse for-mation with host spinal cord (inter)neurons, and termination of transected host axons along grafted neurons.[5] Partial recovery of hindlimb motor function was reported, which was abol-ished after selective ablation of graft-derived neurons, suggesting a relay mechanism under-lying functional recovery. However, animals were not specifically trained; therefore, it is conceivable that the observed gain in hindlimb motor function was a correlate of spasticity rather than the recovery of voluntary motor function. In addition, the loss of movement after re-transection could be attributed to the spinal shock, with transient loss of spasticity rather than relay destruction with consecutive loss of voluntary hindlimb function. In sum-mary, the relay concept is confirmed as a prin-ciple, but remains to be confirmed in a clinically relevant SCI animal model.

A replication study performed by an in-dependent laboratory was able to confirm neuronal differentiation of grafted fetal spinal cord–derived NSC and robust axon outgrowth into the host tissue.[13] However, functional recovery was not observed. In the complete transection model, fibrous rifts within the fetal cell graft were detected, which may have hampered rostrocaudal reconnection, explain-ing the lack of functional recovery. Moreover, in this replication study clusters of grafted cells were found along the meninges remote from the grafting site, raising the concern that grafted cells bear the risk of uncontrolled migration and even tumor formation.

Taken together, NSC grafts derived from a defined developmental stage can regrow and reconnect in the injured adult mammalian spi-nal cord despite the vast expression of myelin and extracellular matrix–associated inhibitory molecules in a worst-case SCI model. These relatively recent findings are highly promis-ing. However, numerous questions have to be addressed in future studies. Do the grafted cells indeed reconnect CNS regions located rostrally and caudally to the lesion site? Even if there is a structural reconnection, does this lead to functionally relevant reconnections? Will NSC transplantation, especially when using induced pluripotent stem cell (iPSC) sources, be safe in the long term?

Cellular Source for Neural Stem Cell Transplantation

Stem cell sources such as bone marrow–derived mesenchymal stem or stromal cells have been widely investigated, but lack the capacity to generate neural cells (neurons, glia) and result in moderate therapeutic effects at best.[14] In principle, NSC can be harvested from the adult CNS[11,15] to allow autologous transplantation. However, adult NSC can only be obtained from CNS biopsies, and they poorly differentiate into neurons after grafting into the injured spinal cord. The most promising sources of NSC are the following:

1. Primary NSC are taken from the fetal spinal cord at a defined developmental stage (e.g., E14 in rats, corresponding to 6 to 10 weeks of gestation in humans); spinal cord fragments are dissected from the fetal spinal cord, and then dissociated, and primary cells are immediately transplanted.
2. Fetal spinal cord–derived cell lines: fragments of fetal spinal cord are dissociated, immortalized, and propagated in culture over many passages to yield nearly unlimited quantities of NSC for transplantation.
3. NSC derived from undifferentiated embryonic cell masses or iPSC: undifferentiated embryonic cells or adult somatic cells (e.g., skin fibroblasts) reprogrammed to be pluripotent will be propagated and differentiated in vitro to become NSC.

Fetal Spinal Cord–Derived Primary Neural Stem Cells

The major advantage of grafting dissociated fetal spinal cord–derived primary NSC without modification/propagation in vitro is that cells of a defined, "naturally" determined developmental stage—not patterned and differentiated through in vitro simulated steps—can be transplanted. It has been shown in rats that only NSC of a defined developmental stage (E14) are capable of growing extensively in the injured adult spinal cord.[5] Without in vitro manipulation, the risk of uncontrolled cell proliferation and tumor formation is much lower. A major drawback is that fetal spinal cord–derived cells have to be obtained from respective donors (abortions) and transported to the transplantation site.[16] Depending on the varying condition of the source material, the quality of the obtained NSC varies. Moreover, for ethical reasons not every country allows exploiting fetal or embryonic NSC sources. Allogenic fetal graft recipients require immunosuppressant treatment to avoid graft rejection. Substantial experience in respect to this stem cell source has been gathered in Parkinson's disease.[16] Currently, a European Union–funded consortium is investigating the feasibility and efficacy of using fetal midbrain–derived cell transplantation to replace dopaminergic neurons in Parkinson disease patients (http://www.transeuro.org.uk).

Fetal Brain or Spinal Cord–Derived Cell Lines

Cell lines derived from fetal brain or spinal cord are also obtained from abortions. However, material from few abortions is sufficient to generate innumerous NSC in a central laboratory, maintaining an identical high standard of quality. Of course, in vitro manipulation required for propagation and differentiation of cells bears the risk of uncontrolled cell growth. Moreover, propagated cells have to be differentiated to yield a certain NSC type at the appropriate developmental stage. Ethical concerns and the necessity of immunosuppressing the graft recipient also apply to fetal NSC lines. Regenerative effects similar to primary fetal spinal cord–derived NSC can be achieved.[17] This approach is currently investigated in a phase I clinical trial (ClinicalTrials.gov identifier NCT01772810), in which four chronic (between

21. Yu J, Vodyanik MA, Smuga-Otto K, et al. Induced pluripotent stem cell lines derived from human somatic cells. Science 2007;318:1917–1920
22. Salewski RP, Eftekharpour E, Fehlings MG. Are induced pluripotent stem cells the future of cell-based regenerative therapies for spinal cord injury? J Cell Physiol 2010;222:515–521
23. Wernig M, Zhao JP, Pruszak J, et al. Neurons derived from reprogrammed fibroblasts functionally integrate into the fetal brain and improve symptoms of rats with Parkinson's disease. Proc Natl Acad Sci U S A 2008;105:5856–5861
24. Miura K, Okada Y, Aoi T, et al. Variation in the safety of induced pluripotent stem cell lines. Nat Biotechnol 2009;27:743–745
25. Ben-David U, Benvenisty N. The tumorigenicity of human embryonic and induced pluripotent stem cells. Nat Rev Cancer 2011;11:268–277
26. Tsuji O, Miura K, Okada Y, et al. Therapeutic potential of appropriately evaluated safe-induced pluripotent stem cells for spinal cord injury. Proc Natl Acad Sci U S A 2010;107:12704–12709
27. Krencik R, Weick JP, Liu Y, Zhang ZJ, Zhang SC. Specification of transplantable astroglial subtypes from human pluripotent stem cells. Nat Biotechnol 2011;29:528–534
28. Stadtfeld M, Nagaya M, Utikal J, Weir G, Hochedlinger K. Induced pluripotent stem cells generated without viral integration. Science 2008;322:945–949
29. Woltjen K, Michael IP, Mohseni P, et al. piggyBac transposition reprograms fibroblasts to induced pluripotent stem cells. Nature 2009;458:766–770
30. Yu J, Hu K, Smuga-Otto K, et al. Human induced pluripotent stem cells free of vector and transgene sequences. Science 2009;324:797–801
31. Pang ZP, Yang N, Vierbuchen T, et al. Induction of human neuronal cells by defined transcription factors. Nature 2011;476:220–223
32. Son EY, Ichida JK, Wainger BJ, et al. Conversion of mouse and human fibroblasts into functional spinal motor neurons. Cell Stem Cell 2011;9:205–218
33. Thier M, Wörsdörfer P, Lakes YB, et al. Direct conversion of fibroblasts into stably expandable neural stem cells. Cell Stem Cell 2012;10:473–479
34. Chanda S, Ang CE, Davila J, et al. Generation of induced neuronal cells by the single reprogramming factor ASCL1. Stem Cell Rev 2014;3:282–296
35. Nori S, Okada Y, Yasuda A, et al. Grafted human-induced pluripotent stem-cell-derived neurospheres promote motor functional recovery after spinal cord injury in mice. Proc Natl Acad Sci U S A 2011;108:16825–16830
36. Hug A, Weidner N. From bench to beside to cure spinal cord injury: lost in translation? Int Rev Neurobiol 2012;106:173–196
37. Keirstead HS, Nistor G, Bernal G, et al. Human embryonic stem cell-derived oligodendrocyte progenitor cell transplants remyelinate and restore locomotion after spinal cord injury. J Neurosci 2005;25:4694–4705
38. Cummings BJ, Uchida N, Tamaki SJ, et al. Human neural stem cells differentiate and promote locomotor recovery in spinal cord-injured mice. Proc Natl Acad Sci U S A 2005;102:14069–14074

11

Strategies to Overcome the Inhibitory Environment of the Spinal Cord

Elizabeth J. Bradbury and Emily R. Burnside

▦ Introduction: The Tissue Environment of the Injured Spinal Cord is Inhibitory to Repair

The developing and immature mammalian central nervous system (CNS) is capable of significant repair and remodeling after injury. However, this ability is lost in adulthood. Despite some initial attempts by injured adult CNS axons to mount a regenerative response, axonal sprouting is abortive, long-distance regeneration does not occur, new connections are not made, and function is lost. An injury to the spinal cord is a particularly powerful example of the debilitating effects of CNS injury, where disruption of long ascending and descending sensory and motor spinal projections can lead to devastating and permanent loss of sensory, motor and autonomic function (**Fig. 11.1**). The poor capacity for repair following CNS injury is in contrast to the adult mammalian peripheral nervous system (PNS), where significant regeneration and functional repair can occur. This raises two questions: What is the difference between the pro-reparative PNS and the unsuccessful CNS? Can we use what we understand about this difference to develop therapeutic concepts to promote repair?

These questions are historic in their origin. In the early 20th century a student of Santiago

Ramón y Cajal performed a cerebral cortex lesion on a rabbit, into which he transplanted a strip of peripheral nerve. Ramón y Cajal described the peripheral nerve transplant to have become occupied by "thick bundles of fibres ... in continuity with the axons of the white and gray matter," detailing the confluence of "newly formed fibres from various points of the cortex, as though they were attracted by an irresistible force."[1] Because these CNS fibers were shown otherwise to have little intrinsic growth potential, the phenomenon inspired the hypothesis that the disparity between PNS and CNS reparative ability could depend on extrinsic environmental factors. Seminal experiments from the laboratories of Aguayo and Richardson explored this concept further, where CNS axons were observed to grow into autologous peripheral (sciatic) nerve graft "bridges" between end-stumps of transected spinal cord,[2] and to possess the ability to elongate long-range through subcutaneously placed grafts between the medulla and spinal cord. Importantly, this unlocked growth-potential was lost when CNS axons were faced with exit from the graft and reentry into the host CNS tissue. Interestingly, if the opposite experiment is performed, in which the sciatic nerve is lesioned and an optic nerve graft inserted, the CNS tissue does not act as a bridge, and regenerating sciatic nerve fibers fail to elongate within the CNS environment.

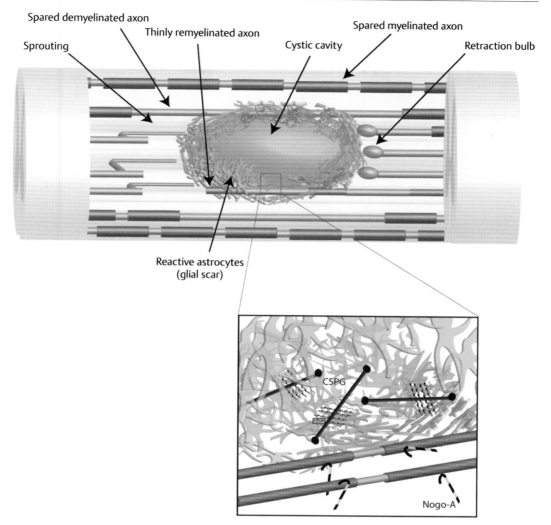

Fig. 11.1 A schematic of the injured spinal cord and its pathological hallmarks. Primary axonal and vascular damage, cell death, increased blood–brain barrier permeability, and the action of proinflammatory cytokines and chemokines lead to glial activation. Reactive astrocytes surround the lesion border and act to seal the blood–brain barrier and spatially isolate spared from damaged tissue. This culminates in glial scar formation around a fluid-filled cystic cavity. Spared axons in the injury penumbra become demyelinated. Injured axons that survive and attempt to regenerate are only thinly myelinated. Retraction bulbs are a feature of failed regenerative responses of axons. Some axons may undergo spontaneous sprouting. However, potent inhibitors present within the spine-injured tissue environment restrict regrowth and repair. **Inset:** Two important examples of growth inhibitors are those associated with myelin (e.g., Nogo-A) and those associated with glial scar extracellular matrix (e.g., chondroitin sulfate proteoglycans [CSPGs]).

Initially, the studies that followed focused on determining what is so permissive about the environment of the PNS. What does the CNS lack that the PNS has? The phenomenon, not dissimilar to that of attractive target-derived growth factors in the developing nervous system, provoked hypotheses centered around specific PNS-derived trophic factors; perhaps the PNS, unlike the CNS, harbored the required growth factors to support repair. However, attempts to mimic the PNS milieu, including exogenous application of growth factors, failed to promote significant ingrowth of sensory fibers into CNS tissue. Indeed, it was the alternative question, What is so nonpermissive about the environment of the CNS? that led to the identification of several inhibitory molecules present in the CNS that actively and potently inhibit neurite outgrowth. These inhibitory molecules have become a major focus of repair strategies, opening a new field of promoting repair by targeting, inhibiting, or neutralizing molecules present in the injured CNS that restrict the potential for growth and neuroplasticity. So, what does the CNS environment have that the PNS environment does not? Here we focus on two major classes of identified growth inhibitors (depicted in **Fig. 11.1**): those associated with CNS myelin and those associated with the extracellular matrix.

▦ Myelin-Associated Inhibitory Molecules

Present in the PNS are myelinating Schwann cells, which are rich in basement membrane, constituents of which are known to be appropriately adhesive and to provide supportive substratum to neurons (such as collagen type IV, fibronectin, and most markedly laminin). Conversely, early in vitro experiments indicated that the myelin from CNS oligodendrocytes contained inhibitory molecules. Plating neurons onto frozen CNS sections revealed maximally myelinated regions to be the poorest substrates for adhesion, survival, and growth; furthermore, white matter extracts from spinal cord, but not sciatic nerve, were inhibitory

to neurite extension. Two membrane protein fractions of 35 and 250 kd purified from spinal cord myelin extracts led to the isolation of what was later identified as Nogo-A, a member of the Reticulon family of proteins (Rtn-4).[3,4] The *Nogo/Rtn4* gene encodes three isoforms (Nogo-A, -B, -C) of which Nogo-A is the largest and the most widely studied, with a wealth of evidence indicating that Nogo-A is a potent growth inhibitor in the injured CNS. Moreover, it has dual inhibitory action on neurons, causing local arrest and collapse of growth cones in addition to retrograde downregulation of neuronal growth programs.[5]

In addition to Nogo-A, myelin-associated glycoprotein (MAG), a single-transmembrane protein expressed both by Schwann cells in the PNS and oligodendrocytes in the CNS, has also been identified as an inhibitor of adult neurons in vitro. Similarly, another protein fraction from CNS myelin, oligodendrocyte myelin glycoprotein (OMgp), inhibits neurite outgrowth in vitro. Nogo-A, MAG, and OMgp all signal via multi-subunit receptor complexes and downstream activation of the canonical RhoA/Rho kinase (ROCK) signaling pathway, which results in destabilization of the actin cytoskeleton and growth cone collapse. However, in vivo evidence for the presence of MAG and OMgp, accounting for the inhibitory properties of the extracellular environment, is lacking. Single, double, or triple knockout mouse studies for Nogo-A, MAG, and OMgp reveal that MAG and OMgp apparently do not limit axonal growth individually, but their deletion may augment the effect of Nogo-A deletion. Other myelin-associated inhibitory molecules include semaphorins, repulsive guidance molecules, and netrins, which, in addition to their axon guidance function in development, are likely to be of some importance in "tuning" plasticity in some regions or specific connections. However, they are not discussed further in this chapter because their overall contribution to inhibition in vivo after injury, relative to other inhibitory components of the environment, is less clear. **Fig. 11.2** depicts the major myelin-associated growth inhibitors and their receptors and signaling pathways. Strategies to intervene at the various protein, receptor, and downstream signaling levels (also depicted in the figure) are discussed later in this chapter.

Extracellular Matrix-Associated Inhibitory Molecules

The extracellular matrix (ECM) provides both a structural framework and an active signaling environment to CNS tissue, the latter occurring both directly via receptor or co-receptor mediated signaling and indirectly via the temporal and spatial localization of other molecules. Moreover, the ECM in the CNS is specialized. It is uniquely rich in glycoproteins and proteoglycans, which may be arranged diffusely in interstitial space or in clustered assemblies around the cell soma of particular neuronal subtypes (perineuronal nets) and also surrounding some synaptic boutons and nodes of Ranvier in the spinal cord. The composition of the adult ECM, including the formation of perineuronal nets, is thought to confer stability following nervous system development-to-purpose, containing molecules that restrict plasticity such as chondroitin sulfate proteoglycans (CSPGs).[6] With regard to an inhibitory CNS environment, the CSPG subtypes most studied include lecticans (aggrecan, versican, neurocan and brevican), the transmembrane protein neural/glial antigen 2 (NG2), phosphacan (transmembrane or soluble), and the small leucine-rich proteoglycans decorin and biglycan. Lecticans are the most abundant and also feature globular domains, the G1 N-terminal domain and G3 C-terminal domains being particularly important in their interaction via link-protein with hyaluronan (the backbone glycoprotein of the CNS matrix) and also tenascin; thus, they are involved in matrix cross-linking and perineuronal net stabilization. All CSPGs are composed of a core protein with at least one covalently attached chondroitin sulfate glycosaminoglycan (CS-GAG) sugar chain.[6] The structure and composition of CSPGs and CS-GAGs are depicted in **Fig. 11.2**.

The CSPGs are upregulated in the extrinsic environment following spinal cord injury (SCI). Injury-induced primary axonal and vascular

damage initiates cascading secondary pathology. Increased blood–brain barrier permeability and the action of proinflammatory cytokines and chemokines leads to glial activation. Most markedly this includes reactive astrocytes, which proliferate and surround the lesion border and change morphology, acting to seal the blood–brain barrier and spatially isolate healthy from damaged tissue (**Fig. 11.1**). Both glia and fibroblast-type cells contribute to the formation of a scar. Though initially protective against secondary damage, substantial and persistent scar-derived matrix is thought to restrict neuroplasticity and repair, largely due to being enriched in CSPGs. Early evidence from in vitro experiments with scar explants and astrocyte cell lines demonstrated that astrocyte-derived CSPGs were neuronal inhibitors, in which neurons were unable to grow on CSPG-rich substrates,[7] an effect mirrored in vivo in situations where CSPG-rich borders were associated with abortive regenerative attempts in the injured spinal cord.[8] Although some core CSPG proteins have been shown to possess inhibitory properties, it is the sulfated CS-GAG chain component that is thought to mediate the largest proportion of inhibition. Because early studies demonstrated that enzymatic removal of CS-GAG using the enzyme chondroitinase ABC (ChABC) in vitro could reverse neurite growth arrest,[7] this has become a major strategy to modify the ECM in experimental SCI studies (discussed below). Furthermore, there is increasing experimental evidence in favor of specific GAG sulfation motifs playing a crucial role in imparting this inhibition, whereby use of pure synthetic GAG structures provides a strong indication that CChondroitin-sulfate E (CS-E) in particular conveys inhibition following CNS injury.[9] Several membrane-bound receptors for CSPGs are now reported to impart neuronal inhibition, all of which are either shared, or share converging downstream signaling pathways, with myelin-associated inhibitors; they are shown in **Fig. 11.2**, along with various experimental strategies to block matrix-associated inhibitors.

This chapter discusses experimental approaches that have attempted to overcome inhibitory factors present in the injured adult mammalian CNS as a strategy to promote

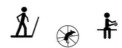

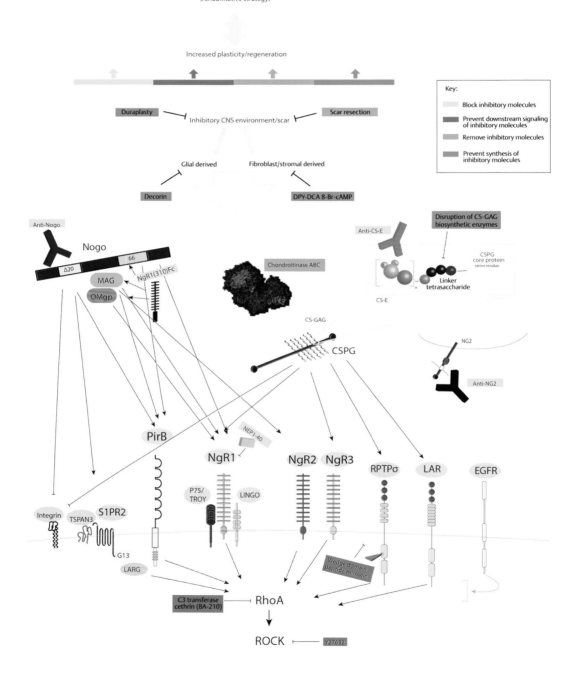

Fig. 11.2 (*opposite*) Identified growth inhibitors associated with central nervous system (CNS) myelin and glial scar extracellular matrix associated in the injured spinal cord environment. The schematic depicts both the interaction of environmental inhibitors with their respective effectors, and four categories of experimental strategies designed to overcome this interaction: strategies that block binding of inhibitors to their functional receptor, strategies that prevent downstream signaling, strategies that remove inhibitors from the environment, and strategies that prevent their biosynthesis (depicted in *yellow, blue, orange,* and *green,* respectively). For simplicity only the most relevant interactions are depicted schematically, but others are cited in this legend. *Myelin-associated inhibitors*: two Nogo domains are implicated in imparting inhibition: Nogo-66 and Nogo-A-Δ20. Nogo-66 is a 66-amino-acid residue extracellular loop between two transmembrane portions of the protein, a component of the Reticulon (Rtn) homology domain, which is present in the C-terminus of all Nogo isoforms. Receptors include Nogo Receptor 1 (NgR1), forming a transmembrane complex with a leucine rich repeat and immunoglobin-like domain-containing protein (LINGO) or one member of the tumor necrosis factor receptor superfamily (TROY), and it can also signal via the paired immunoglobulin-like receptor B (PirB) in some cell types. Nogo-A-Δ20 inhibition occurs via its functional receptor sphingosine 1-phosphate receptor 2 (S1PR2) and modulatory co-receptor four-transmembrane-spanning protein tetraspanin-3 (TSPAN3), which is additionally thought to mediate retrograde downregulation of nuclear growth programs. Its activity is also partially mediated by integrin inhibition. Signaling of both functional receptors converges on the canonical RhoA/Rho kinase (ROCK) signaling pathway, resulting in destabilization of the actin cytoskeleton. Oligodendrocyte myelin glycoprotein (OMgp) also binds NgR1, and there are multiple functional receptors for myelin-associated glycoprotein (MAG): NgR1, NgR2, and PirB, and also gangliosides GD1a and GT1b, β1-integrin, and pancreatic lipase-related protein 1 (LIPR1) (not shown). *Extracellular matrix-associated inhibitors (CSPGs)*: membrane-bound receptors reported to impart CSPG-mediated neuronal inhibition include receptor *protein tyrosine phosphatase-σ* (RPTPσ), leukocyte common antigen-related phosphatase (LAR), and NgR1 and NgR3. Signaling pathways implicated again include the Rho/ROCK pathway, activation of which is also partly via protein kinase C (PKC) and epidermal growth factor receptor (EGFR) and coupled to Akt/Glycogen synthase kinase 3 (GSK-3) activation (not depicted). Like Nogo, CSPGs are also thought to inactivate neural integrins. Chondroitin sulfate glycosaminoglycans (CS-GAGs) are repeating disaccharide units attached to the core protein via a tetrasaccharide link to form a long linear polysaccharide chain. Sulfation motifs are additionally thought to confer particular interactive properties. DPY-DCA, 2,2′dipyridine-5,5′-dicarboxylic acid; NG2, neural/glial antigen 2.

repair and restore function after SCI. Most of these approaches target either myelin-associated or ECM-associated inhibitors. Here we consider these strategies in terms of the therapeutic approach. We discuss the following: (1) approaches that have attempted to mask or block functional receptor binding of inhibitory molecules (e.g., with the use of neutralizing antibodies); (2) strategies to prevent their downstream signaling (e.g., by inhibiting effector molecules); (3) approaches to remove CNS inhibitors altogether from the environment (e.g., with enzymatic degradation); and (4) strategies to prevent the initial accumulation of these inhibitors by blocking them at the stage of synthesis (e.g., by inhibiting biosynthetic enzymes). These strategies are summarized in **Fig. 11.2**, with the four approaches depicted in yellow, blue, orange, and green, respectively. Finally, we touch on the importance of consolidating these approaches, whereby regeneration or neuroplasticity-promoting treatments can be combined with targeted rehabilitation to direct and consolidate appropriate connections and promote useful recovery of function.

Masking or Blocking Inhibitory Molecules

Antibodies to Mask Inhibitory Factors

Blocking interactive or functional domains of known inhibitory molecules with antibodies is one experimental strategy to overcome their presence in the extracellular environment (highlighted in *yellow* in **Fig. 11.2**). Neutralizing Nogo-A represents a leading translational endeavor in blocking myelin-associated inhibition following SCI.[5] In studies dating back to the 1990s, application of IN-1, an immunoglobulin M (IgM) recognizing the Nogo-A specific domain (Nogo-A-Δ20), increased neural regeneration in the injured adult rat spinal cord, leading to functional sensorimotor improvement. Similar effects were observed with two immunoglobulin G (IgG) antibodies also raised against Nogo-A-Δ20, and these were also found to internalize bound Nogo-A, acting to downregulate endogenous levels of the inhibitory protein.[3] Numerous studies have since demonstrated functional regeneration and rewiring of spinal and supraspinal systems following experimental SCI and intrathecally delivered anti-Nogo in both rodent and nonhuman primates.[5]

Moving toward clinical trial, a humanized version of anti-Nogo (ATI355) was synthesized in collaboration with Novartis. In adult macaque monkeys, intrathecal administration of ATI355 mediated regeneration of corticospinal axons and recovery of precision grip following cervical spinal injury.[10] A phase I/II open label, no controls, study of ATI355 involved 52 acutely injured American Spinal Injury Association (ASIA) grade A paraplegic and tetraplegic patients, with treatment starting 5 to 21 days following injury. Initially, anti-Nogo was delivered via intrathecal pump; however, to avoid potential risks related to invasive catheter placement, subsequent dosing used six repeated intrathecal injections over 30 days, based on pharmacokinetic data obtained during initial stages of the trial. Exposure and dose escalation data demonstrated the safety of ATI355, with no reported side effects.[5,11] A phase II trial is now in preparation, sponsored by the Horizon 2020 EU Program. It is expected to recruit patients beginning in 2016, using an unbiased recursive partitioning strategy to stratify 158 patients in a manner that overcomes the problems heterogeneous injury populations impose on statistically powerful trial design. Alongside clinical monitoring and pharmacovigilance, the trial is expected to provide additional valu-

able data collection that, for example, could inform biomarker studies. It is hoped that this sophisticated design could serve as a template for future translation of other promising therapeutic strategies.

Antibodies have also been used to target inhibitory CSPGs. A function-blocking antibody to NG2, for example, had moderate effects on neural sprouting in several studies but more robust benefits in improving axonal conduction and function following intraspinal injection after hemisection injury.[12] Furthermore, in an advancement in understanding the role of particular CS-GAG sulfation patterns, antibodies have also been generated to specific CS-GAG sulfation motifs, where an anti-CS-E was shown to reverse CSPG inhibition in vitro and promote regeneration in vivo following optic nerve crush.[9] If CS-E does indeed represent the major inhibitory determinant of CSPGs, this refined strategy to target CSPGs may benefit approaches to overcome inhibition of plasticity. More research is needed as to whether this would outweigh the multiple beneficial effects that have been observed with a more global method of removing all forms of sulfated GAGs with the enzyme ChABC (discussed in more detail below), but one can envisage temporal and spatial considerations that could render both strategies complementary in overcoming the negative aspects of CSPGs following injury.

Manipulating Functional Receptors of Inhibitory Factors

In addition to antibody-mediated approaches to target the inhibitory ligand, preventing action of the ligand by antagonizing its binding to its functional receptor represents another method of blocking environmental inhibition (highlighted in *yellow* in **Fig. 11.2**). For example, a Nogo-66 receptor antagonist NEP1–40 was developed as a strategy to block inhibitory myelin receptor binding to this functional receptor and showed some promise in experimental animals with spinal hemisection injuries, although these effects were not always fully replicated. A more recent approach to block Nogo Receptor 1 (NgR1) has shown impressive effects in preclinical studies. A soluble NgR1 decoy protein consisting of the ectodomain of NgR1 fused to an IgG incapable of signal transduction (NgR1(310)-Fc, Axerion Therapeutics, Branford, CT) has shown efficacy in clinically relevant rodent contusion injuries, with both acute and chronic administration resulting in functional improvements.[13] Moreover, pharmacokinetic studies in rats and nonhuman primates suggest bolus lumbar infusion via lumbar puncture to be as effective as constant infusion via indwelling catheter, and a clinical trial using NgR1(310)-Fc is being planned for the near future.[5]

This approach complements the antibody strategy to target Nogo-A, as although both Nogo-66 and Nogo-A-Δ20 are thought to converge on the same signaling and cytoskeletal effectors, they have non-overlapping receptor binding profiles. Anti-Nogo targets Nogo-A-Δ20, whereas NgR1(310)-Fc prevents action of Nogo-66. Furthermore, NgR1(310)-Fc also binds OMgp and MAG. Of relevance, although CSPGs bind to NgR1, CSPG inhibition is not overcome alone by NgR1 knockout, as it acts via multiple receptors, but this approach may also have some effect on CSPG signaling.

Preventing Downstream Signaling of Inhibitory Factors

Preventing communication between the functional receptor of an inhibitory ligand and its downstream effectors represents another strategy to manipulate extrinsic environmental inhibitors (highlighted in *blue* in **Fig. 11.2**). Targeted modulation of CSPG receptor signaling has proved successful via manipulation of the receptor *protein tyrosine phosphatase-σ* (PTPσ). The activity of the intracellular phosphatase domains of PTPσ are regulated via a conserved "wedge" structure that can occlude the catalytic domain, thus reducing phosphorylatory activity and ability to signal downstream. Use of a membrane-permeable peptide mimetic of this wedge reduces PTPσ signaling following activation by ligands such as CSPGs, and systemic delivery of this peptide has been shown to promote functional recovery of locomotor

and urinary systems in rats with spinal contusion injuries[14] and represents a promising therapeutic approach.

Effectors of CSPG inhibition are also thought to be influenced by epidermal growth factor (EGF) signaling pathways, and there is evidence that inhibiting downstream mitogen-activated protein kinase (MAPK) or blocking the kinase activity of the EGF receptor (EGFR) can significantly reduce CSPG-mediated inhibition. Competitive or nonreversible inhibition of EGFR signaling with well-characterized small molecule inhibitors was shown to promote repair in an optic nerve crush model and to improve sensorimotor and bladder functions following weight-drop contusion injury.[15] Although this effect has not yet been replicated, the approach of repurposing drugs already in clinical use for other indications, to target signaling pathways known to inhibit growth and repair, represents an important route to discovering new therapeutics for SCI.

The convergence of known extrinsic inhibitor signaling on the Rho/ROCK pathway is attractive to therapeutic manipulation. In addition to roles in other cell types, the pathway is canonical to neural inhibition. The Rho family of guanosine triphosphatases (GTPases) regulates cytoskeletal dynamics downstream of almost every axon guidance signaling pathway and known extrinsic inhibitory molecule following injury. Regulated by guanine nucleotide-exchange factors (GEFs) and GTPase activating proteins (GAPs), the pathway enables spatial control of actin dynamics and coordination of microtubule cross-linking, physical processes underlying neural attraction or inhibition. Inhibition of the Rho/ROCK pathway has resulted in promising in vivo effects in two well-studied experimental paradigms: injections of C3 transferase to inactivate Rho, and small catalytic site inhibitors of ROCK (depicted in *blue* in **Fig. 11.2**).

C3 transferase is an enzyme from *Clostridium botulinum* that catalyses adenosine diphosphate (ADP)-ribosylation of Rho, a modification that maintains it in an inactive state. Following robust in vitro effects on neurite outgrowth and optic nerve regeneration models with this enzyme, a membrane-permeable recombinant protein form of this rho inhibitor, Cethrin (BA-210), was synthesized, which permeates the entire rodent spinal cord. This had promising effects on functional locomotor recovery following experimental thoracic contusion and partial transection of the spinal cord.[16] Following this positive preclinical data, Cethrin has been utilized in an open label phase I/IIa multicenter trial in 48 thoracic and cervical spine injured ASIA patients, in which a single dose of Cethrin was topically applied in fibrin sealant extradurally during acute surgical intervention following injury. Cethrin was found to be safe, and clinical trials are ongoing toward assessment of efficacy with placebo control. Published comparative assessments to historical natural expected recovery data (retrospective longitudinal information derived from the Sygen Multicenter Acute Spinal Cord Injury Study and the European Multicenter Study of Spinal Cord Injury [EMSCI]) suggest some trends to improvement,[17] and a phase II/III randomized controlled trial of Cethrin in patients with severe cervical SCI has recently been initiated, sponsored by Vertex Pharmaceuticals (Boston, MA). ROCK is a serine threonine kinase downstream effector of RhoA. Following promising in vitro and optic nerve regeneration data, inhibition of ROCK has been achieved in SCI studies by intrathecal delivery of the inhibitor Y-27632, which promoted corticospinal tract regeneration and accelerated early stages of recovery.[18] Fasudil, another potent ROCK inhibitor (and vasodilator), and KD025, a ROCKII subtype-specific inhibitor, have also been utilized with positive experimental findings, although the number of reported studies remains low. A meta-analysis of all preclinical Rho/ROCK manipulation strategies concludes that publication bias is significant in this area of experimental study, but that after accounting for this bias, a 15% effect size in functional improvement would still be expected.[19] Therefore, although small trends to improvement in the Cethrin phase I/IIa trial in only 48 patients must be interpreted with caution, and this presents a challenge to ongoing trials to achieve statistical power, a 15% improvement in outcome would be of significant clinical relevance.

■ Removing Inhibitory Molecules

On a surgical scale, resection of scar tissue represents a gross-level approach to eliminate inhibitory tissue. Scar resection has been utilized occasionally in chronic preclinical and clinical research interventions, usually prior to bridging or transplantation surgery. However, there are obvious technical challenges in removing tissue without risking the loss of the remaining function. Instead, most experimental strategies are chemically focused for proteolysis of defined targets (strategies to remove inhibitory molecules are highlighted in *orange* in **Fig. 11.2**).

Strategies to Break Down Scar Tissue

Early proteolytic strategies to break down scar tissue included trypsin, hyaluronidase, and elastase administration following experimental spinal transection, but such harsh approaches can also degrade vascular membranes and cause hemorrhage. Endogenous extracellular proteases are present in the CNS. These remodeling enzymes include matrix metalloproteinases (MMPs) and the ADAM (a disintegrin and metalloprotease)/ADAMTS (a disintegrin and metalloprotease with thrombospondin motifs) families, which collectively have the potential to degrade most protein components within the ECM, including inhibitory molecules and receptors for inhibitory cues. They are involved in injury and in both beneficial and detrimental repair mechanisms. Studies have attempted to harness some enzymes in this tightly regulated network. In particular, intrathecal delivery of ADAMTS-4 was shown to attenuate CSPG inhibition and promote functional recovery in adult rats with spinal contusions.[20] Given that ADAMTS-4 is an endogenous mammalian enzyme, this strategy represents a promising avenue for further investigation.

Chondroitinase ABC

The most common strategy to remove inhibitory molecules from the CNS environment is use of the bacterial enzyme chondroitinase ABC (ChABC). ChABC represents one of the most promising preclinical treatments for SCI, having shown robust and replicable beneficial effects across multiple laboratories, in different species and CNS injury models.[21] Following in vitro evidence that ChABC treatment rendered inhibitory substrates growth-permissive[7] and in vivo confirmation that ChABC was able to degrade CNS injury-derived CSPGs and promote axonal regeneration in the brain,[22] it was shown for the first time in 2002 that ChABC treatment could result in functional improvements following SCI in adult rats.[23] Studies that followed have replicated the beneficial effects of ChABC, as well as elucidated the mechanisms behind functional improvements and also considered dose, timing, and method of delivery.

With the exception of approaches that are currently in clinical trials, or in preparation for clinical trial, ChABC has generated the most significant preclinical body of evidence of efficacy of any potential therapeutic that aims to overcome the inhibitory environment of the spinal cord following injury. Alongside increasing plasticity and functional repair following brain and peripheral nerve injury, ChABC has conferred benefit in a range of experimental SCI models. Numerous beneficial effects of ChABC treatment have been reported in partial injury studies, including regeneration, neuroplasticity, neuroprotection, and immune modulation.[24] Such immunomodulatory and neuroprotective effects culminate in the generation of a less inhibitory environment as well increasing the number of cells that are viable and thus amenable to harnessing this less inhibitory environment. Ensuing studies have also established significant functional benefit in clinically relevant contusive-type injury models,[25,26] a promising step toward clinical translation of this approach. Additionally, intrathecal administration has proved beneficial in larger animal spinal injury models including rabbits, pigs, and cats.[21] Moreover, ChABC has proved to be a useful strategy to combine with other therapeutic interventions, rendering the environment permissive to enable cell transplant graft integration or reentry of fibers growing through permissive grafts into the CNS with significant improvements observed, including restoration of bladder function.[27]

With regard to delivery of ChABC, following administration of the unmodified enzyme, activity is thought to diminish within a week and CS-GAGs are thought to remodel within 2 to 3 weeks. Thus, single-injection administration has limited beneficial effect following CNS trauma. Sustained environmental matrix modification would therefore necessitate repeated invasive administrations, which poses a challenge for clinical translation. Attempts to overcome this include a trehalose-thermostabilized modified enzyme, which enables slow-release activity for up to a month, promoting functional recovery following a partial transection injury[28] and leading to its use in a canine "clinical trial" study. Alternatively, a gene therapy approach circumvents the need for repeated injection or biocarrier, whereby host cells are transduced to synthesize ChABC themselves following intraparenchymal injection. This strategy, using a modified ChABC gene with optimal properties for release from mammalian cells, has enabled extensive long-term matrix modification, promoting improved axonal conduction and functional recovery in clinically relevant thoracic and cervical contusion injuries in adult rats.[26,29] Thus, chondroitinase gene therapy shows great promise for future clinical development. To this end, the Chondroitinase ABC for Spinal Injury Therapy (CHASE-IT) consortium has been established to pursue the development of a regulatable and safe vector for future human use (http://www.spinal-research.org/chondroitinase).

An alternative enzymatic strategy that has recently been exploited for reducing CSPG inhibition is the mammalian enzyme arylsulfatase B (ARSB, N-acetylgalatosamine-4-sulfatase), which removes C4S moieties specifically from CS-GAGs. In addition to being utilized in enzyme-replacement therapy for human mucopolysaccharidosis VI, ARSB administration has been shown in one study to promote increased axonal sprouting and functional locomotor recovery following compression SCI in the mouse,[30] and this promising approach certainly warrants further investigation.

Targeting Synthesis of Inhibitory Factors

Targeting the synthesis of inhibitory factors after SCI can be viewed on two levels. The first is broadly reducing the synthesis of scar matrix, which is known to contain multiple inhibitory molecules. The second is to target upregulation of specific molecules themselves within the scar environment. (Strategies to target the synthesis of inhibitory factors are highlighted in *green* in **Fig. 11.2.**)

Strategies to Reduce Synthesis of Scar Tissue

On a surgical scale, apposition and suturing of severed dura and optional patching with another soft tissue material (duraplasty) is suggested to limit fibrotic and connective tissue deposition from meningeal-derived fibroblasts. Additionally, removal of dura following experimental spinal contusion injury (which normally leaves the dura intact) results in increased scar formation (and lesion volume and inflammatory response), whereas decompressive durotomy followed by dural allograft has been shown to reduce scar formation relative to contusion alone (and improve lesion volume and inflammatory response).[31]

A particular pharmacological approach designed to suppress formation of the scar following injury is often termed anti-scarring treatment (AST). The best studied example of this is injections or slow release of local iron chelator 2,2′dipyridine-5,5′-dicarboxylic acid (DPY-DCA) combined with solid 8-bromocyclic adenosine monophosphate (8-Br-cAMP) application to the lesion core by injection. DPY-DCA deprives a key enzyme in the synthesis of all types of collagen (prolyl 4-hydroxylase) of its cofactor ion, and 8-Br-cAMP inhibits meningeal fibroblast proliferation, with the collective effect of reducing the formation of fibrotic scar matrix capable of presenting inhibitory

molecules such as CSPGs.[32] Additionally, a clinically approved ion chelator deferoxamine mesylate (DFO) can reduce fibrotic scarring with moderate anatomic and functional benefits, and inhibition of lysyl oxidase, another key collagen biosynthetic enzyme, can also mediate functional effects, after partial spinal transection. Less well studied is whether it is also effective in inhibiting fibroblast-derived matrix synthesis following a contusive-type injury, where the dura is intact and the composition of *meningeal* fibroblastic deposition has been thought to be of less significance than glial scar deposition. However, given that type I collagen has been identified in rat contusion injuries around blood vessels, and that some human contusive injuries feature a dense fibrotic matrix,[33] inhibition of collagen synthesis (whether fibrillar type I or basement membrane laminar IV) could represent a conserved mechanism to broadly reduce formation of a fibroblast-type cell-derived scar matrix, following both penetrative and contusive spinal injury.

Another experimental method to suppress scar formation is administration of the small leucine-rich proteoglycan decorin. Decorin binds to the cytokine transforming growth factor- (TGF-β), resulting in inhibition of injury-induced TGF-β1/2 signaling. Following SCI, TGF-β1/2 is released from multiple cell types with multiple effects. Notably initial expression by extravasated platelets induces reactive gliosis and accompanied matrix deposition. This is reduced by decorin core protein administration following dorsal funicular lesions by reducing glial activation, inflammation, and synthesis of known inhibitory scar molecules such as CSPGs.[34,35] However, this treatment alone is of limited functional outcome or benefit. The concept underlying strategies attenuating *glial* scar synthesis is that the initial glial scar is protective. Following injury, reactive astrocytes actively engage in an orchestrated wound-healing response. In vivo premature attenuation or prevention of glial scar formation can result in delayed blood–brain barrier closure, exacerbated lesion spread, neuronal loss, and reduced functional recovery. For this reason another strategy is to specifically target the synthesis of inhibitory constituents of the glial scar matrix rather than its presence as a whole.

Targeting Synthesis of Specific Environment Inhibitors

The CSPGs are upregulated in the glial scar, whereby GAG chains are thought to mediate a large proportion of inhibition. A specific biosynthetic strategy is to interrupt GAG chain synthesis, without primary effect on the rest of the matrix. There are multiple CS-GAG biosynthetic enzymes. One approach has been to inhibit xylotransferase-1, the enzyme that catalyses GAG addition to the CSPG core protein, by deoxyribozyme-mediated knockdown of xylosyltransferase-1 messenger RNA (mRNA). This approach has resulted in significant improvement in axon growth into scarred tissue around a peripheral nerve graft, axonal sprouting caudal to the injury, and some functional sensorimotor improvement following spinal contusion injury.[36]

Having shown via gain and loss of function experiments in vitro that xylosyltransferase enzymes I and II alongside chondroitin-4-sulfotransferase (C4ST) are part of a group of genes regulated upstream by sox9, conditional sox9 ablation in mice has been shown to reduce CSPG synthesis, increase axonal sprouting, and improve functional motor scores after spinal contusion,[37] suggesting that sox9 manipulation could provide a therapeutic avenue to interrupt GAG synthesis. Furthermore, mice lacking chondroitin sulfate N-acetylegalactosaminyl-transferase-1, the enzyme that catalyses the addition of the first GalNAc residue onto the tetrasaccharide link between the core proteoglycan (PG) and GAG (and thus is rate-limiting to GAG formation), synthesize less CS-GAGs into the scar matrix following contusion injury and show better functional recovery relative to wild-type controls. Interestingly, knockout of the enzyme not only reduced CS but increased heparan sulfate synthesis, which conferred significant additional benefit to axonal growth,[38] in accordance with the known growth-promoting role of heparan sulfate following injury. Mechanistic questions remain, but inhibition of this particular GAG biosynthetic enzyme seems to both prevent synthesis of inhibitory factors into the environment and promote intrinsic growth.

Toward increasing levels of specificity in targeting synthesis of CSPGs as a strategy to overcome CNS growth inhibition, studies have begun to address inhibiting sulfotransferases to target synthesis of specific CS-GAG sulfation epitopes. CSPGs isolated from knockout mice for the sulfotransferase that synthesizes CS-E (GalNAc4S-6ST) are less inhibitory, as are CSPGs synthesized from astrocytes in which GalNAc4S-6ST or C4ST are knocked-down using small double-stranded interfering RNA (siRNA). Given success in inhibition of such sulfotransferases among other enzymes in vivo,[37] and the increasing evidence that these sulfation patterns play specific roles in the scar matrix,[9] this represents an interesting avenue of future work. The complement DNA (cDNA) of the genes encoding GAG biosynthetic enzymes are now cloned (from genetic GAG biosynthetic enzyme deficiency disorders). Based on this knowledge and the aforementioned in vitro and in vivo knockdown/knockout studies, progression from knockout mice to pharmacological inhibition of biosynthetic enzymes will be an important next step for the generation of therapeutically applicable interventions aimed at overcoming growth inhibition in the injured spinal cord.

Making the Most of a Permissive Environment: Consolidating Environmental Changes to Promote Functional Repair

Rendering the extracellular environment permissive to neuroplasticity lacks benefit if plasticity cannot be usefully harnessed. Therefore, strategies to overcome the inhibitory environment of the CNS also require the generation of functionally useful connectivity. It is possible that strategies to overcome the inhibitory environment of the spinal cord may require a combination of approaches to boost intrinsic growth capability, for example, to enable axons to take greater advantage of a permissive environment, but crucially, consolidation of the correct kind of plasticity is a universal consideration. Learned non-use is a major impediment to recovery, and rehabilitation is an important means to offer input and sensory feedback to the nervous system to promote, train, and refine connectivity. Indeed, the inclusion of precisely timed electrophysiological stimulation within a rehabilitative strategy to strengthen connectivity in line with both appropriate sensory input/feedback and desired motor output is one approach designed to facilitate this further. Additionally, anatomic reorganization does not always equal functional recovery, and the concept of maladaptive plasticity is particularly important when promoting neural rewiring.

Timing of rehabilitation is a critical factor in promoting functional recovery. Despite limited plasticity in the adult CNS, there is a phase of spontaneous regrowth that is thought to be best targeted by therapeutic strategies that aim to overcome the inhibitory environment and act to increase plasticity. Training and rehabilitation should be coordinated with, or follow, this plastic phase to shape novel circuitry to maximize functional use. Additionally, there is evidence that rehabilitative strategies that begin too early may be detrimental. In a study in which rats with cervical spinal lesions were treated intrathecally with anti-Nogo and received daily bipedal step training for 8 weeks beginning 1 week postinjury, simultaneous therapy worsened functional outcome relative to either strategy alone.[39] However, the delay of forced treadmill training until 2 weeks following cessation of antibody treatment led to significant improvement in functional recovery.[40]

In addition, task-specificity is a well-documented feature of functional recovery in rehabilitation regimes. Following intense training, adult spinalized cats can be trained either to step on a treadmill or to bear weight bear while remaining stationary. Cats trained to step do not recover weight-bearing standing, and those trained to bear weight bear cannot step on a treadmill. Thus, in addition to reflecting a high level of automaticity in some spinal systems (known to be dependent on correct sensory feedback), specific activation of spinal circuitry reinforces specific connectivity. Similarly, fine-skilled reaching training for 6 weeks in rats following unilateral cervical lesion improved success in this task, but came at the detriment of motor function in the form of ladder walking relative to untrained rats.[41] Importantly, further work from this group extinguished this negative transfer effect on performance by delaying the onset of skilled rehabilitation. Crucially, this phenomenon also extends to experimental studies in which the inhibitory environment of the spinal cord is ameliorated, and plasticity is therapeutically promoted alongside rehabilitation. Although a group of rats receiving ChABC and manual dexterity training showed functional improvements following cervical dorsal funiculus lesion, general locomotor training in another experimental group of animals worsened their dexterity performance.[42] However, with correct task-specific rehabilitation, this approach is effective even if ChABC is administered 4 weeks following injury,[43] exemplifying the importance of the correct rehabilitation strategy.

Following therapeutic promotion of neuroplasticity and intensive appropriate training, consolidation may require the return of a relatively stable nervous system once connectivity has been established, enabling maintenance and strengthening of optimal connections and "pruning" of those less useful. This has particular relevance to gene therapy–mediated strategies that sustain the expression of therapeutically advantageous proteins. An important aim of the CHASE-IT consortium is therefore to develop regulatable systems to allow "switching-off" of treatment when desired.[24]

▪ Chapter Summary

Spinal cord injury results in permanent and debilitating motor, sensory, and autonomic deficits. With patients facing a lifetime of disability and no adequate treatments available, there is a clear clinical requirement for therapeutic developments. The adult CNS has a poor ability to repair itself following SCI, in contrast to the pro-regenerative adult PNS. Such comparison inspired experimental investigations that identified factors other than neuronal intrinsic determinants to be crucial mediators of this phenomenon and led to a major focus on targeting inhibitory factors present in the injured tissue environment that restrict axonal growth and neuroplasticity and limit the potential for spinal cord repair. A notable example is the presence of potent growth inhibitory molecules associated with CNS myelin.

The injured spinal cord extracellular scar matrix is another important mediator of environmental inhibition, and matrix modification to enhance neuroplasticity has also become a major target for repair. Accordingly, in this chapter we considered four different levels of therapeutic strategies that target an inhibitory environment to promote repair following SCI: (1) masking or blocking inhibitory molecules, (2) interrupting their (often converging) downstream signaling, (3) removing them from the environment, and (4) preventing their initial biosynthesis following injury. Some of these strategies are relatively novel, and some possess a wealth of experimental background. Efficacy of a particular antibody-mediated strategy to mask the myelin-associated growth inhibitory molecule Nogo-A has been confirmed in several studies in both rodents and primates, with clear preclinical understanding of its mechanism of action, leading to successful conversion of experimental findings to ongoing clinical trials in patients with acute SCI. Proteolytic breakdown of inhibitory scar matrix by the enzyme ChABC has a large body of preclinical evidence as to its efficacy in a range of experimental spinal injury models and species, and thus represents a leading candidate for translational advance. Cethrin is another important example, because it inhibits downstream signaling of multiple environmental inhibitors (both myelin-associated and scar-associated)

via canonical RhoA/ROCK pathway inhibition, and is currently in clinical trials. Furthermore, the efficacy of all strategies that aim to overcome inhibition in the spinal cord depends on the consolidation of therapeutically promoted neural growth toward functionally useful connectivity. This necessitates avoidance of maladaptive plasticity and a rehabilitative strategy that takes into consideration both timing and the concept of task-dependent rehabilitative recovery.

Pearls

- ◆ Growth inhibitors present in spine-injured tissue represent an important target for regenerative therapies aimed at promoting neuroplasticity and functional repair following SCI.
- ◆ Strategies to neutralize myelin-associated inhibitors are a promising route to increasing neuroplasticity and restoring function following SCI.
- ◆ Strategies to modify inhibitory extracellular matrix molecules are a promising route to increasing neuroplasticity and restoring function following SCI.
- ◆ Strategies targeting environmental inhibitors should be combined with rehabilitation therapy to direct and refine new connections and lead to meaningful functional recovery.
- ◆ Advances in preclinical experimental studies of environmental inhibitors have resulted in several promising therapies progressing to clinical trials in spine-injured patients.

Pitfalls

- ◆ If newly growing axons do not make meaningful connections, function will not be restored.
- ◆ Undirected or misdirected neuronal growth could lead to maladaptive plasticity.
- ◆ The timing of treatment intervention and rehabilitative therapy needs to be carefully considered to avoid conflicting and adverse effects on functional recovery.
- ◆ Statistically powerful trial design is important to avoid misinterpretation of SCI clinical trial data.

References
Five Must-Read References

1. Ramón y Cajal S. Degeneration and Regeneration in the Nervous System. London: Oxford University Press; 1928
2. Richardson PM, McGuinness UM, Aguayo AJ. Axons from CNS neurons regenerate into PNS grafts. Nature 1980;284:264–265
3. Caroni P, Schwab ME. Antibody against myelin-associated inhibitor of neurite growth neutralizes non-permissive substrate properties of CNS white matter. Neuron 1988;1:85–96
4. Goldberg JL, Barres BA. Nogo in nerve regeneration. Nature 2000;403:369–370
5. Schwab ME, Strittmatter SM. Nogo limits neural plasticity and recovery from injury. Curr Opin Neurobiol 2014;27:53–60
6. Burnside ER, Bradbury EJ. Manipulating the extracellular matrix and its role in brain and spinal cord plasticity and repair. Neuropathol Appl Neurobiol 2014;40:26–59
7. Smith-Thomas LC, Fok-Seang J, Stevens J, et al. An inhibitor of neurite outgrowth produced by astrocytes. J Cell Sci 1994;107(Pt 6):1687–1695
8. Davies SJ, Goucher DR, Doller C, Silver J. Robust regeneration of adult sensory axons in degenerating white matter of the adult rat spinal cord. J Neurosci 1999;19:5810–5822
9. Brown JM, Xia J, Zhuang B, et al. A sulfated carbohydrate epitope inhibits axon regeneration after injury. Proc Natl Acad Sci U S A 2012;109:4768–4773
10. Freund P, Schmidlin E, Wannier T, et al. Nogo-A-specific antibody treatment enhances sprouting and functional recovery after cervical lesion in adult primates. Nat Med 2006;12:790–792
11. Zörner B, Schwab ME. Anti-Nogo on the go: from animal models to a clinical trial. Ann N Y Acad Sci 2010;1198(Suppl 1):E22–E34
12. Petrosyan HA, Hunanyan AS, Alessi V, Schnell L, Levine J, Arvanian VL. Neutralization of inhibitory molecule NG2 improves synaptic transmission, retrograde transport, and locomotor function after spinal cord injury in adult rats. J Neurosci 2013;33:4032–4043
13. Wang X, Duffy P, McGee AW, et al. Recovery from chronic spinal cord contusion after Nogo receptor intervention. Ann Neurol 2011;70:805–821
14. Lang BT, Cregg JM, DePaul MA, et al. Modulation of the proteoglycan receptor PTPs promotes recovery after spinal cord injury. Nature 2015;518:404–408
15. Erschbamer M, Pernold K, Olson L. Inhibiting epidermal growth factor receptor improves structural, locomotor, sensory, and bladder recovery from experimental spinal cord injury. J Neurosci 2007;27:6428–6435
16. Lord-Fontaine S, Yang F, Diep Q, et al. Local inhibition of Rho signaling by cell-permeable recombinant protein BA-210 prevents secondary damage and promotes functional recovery following acute spinal cord injury. J Neurotrauma 2008;25:1309–1322
17. Fehlings MG, Theodore N, Harrop J, et al. A phase I/IIa clinical trial of a recombinant Rho protein antagonist in acute spinal cord injury. J Neurotrauma 2011;28:787–796
18. Fournier AE, Takizawa BT, Strittmatter SM. Rho kinase inhibition enhances axonal regeneration in the injured CNS. J Neurosci 2003;23:1416–1423
19. Watzlawick R, Sena ES, Dirnagl U, et al. Effect and reporting bias of RhoA/ROCK-blockade intervention on locomotor recovery after spinal cord injury: a systematic review and meta-analysis. JAMA Neurol 2014;71:91–99
20. Tauchi R, Imagama S, Natori T, et al. The endogenous proteoglycan-degrading enzyme ADAMTS-4 promotes functional recovery after spinal cord injury. J Neuroinflammation 2012;9:53
21. Bradbury EJ, Carter LM. Manipulating the glial scar: chondroitinase ABC as a therapy for spinal cord injury. Brain Res Bull 2011;84:306–316
22. Moon LD, Asher RA, Rhodes KE, Fawcett JW. Regeneration of CNS axons back to their target following treatment of adult rat brain with chondroitinase ABC. Nat Neurosci 2001;4:465–466
23. Bradbury EJ, Moon LD, Popat RJ, et al. Chondroitinase ABC promotes functional recovery after spinal cord injury. Nature 2002;416:636–640
24. Ramer LM, Ramer MS, Bradbury EJ. Restoring function after spinal cord injury: towards clinical translation of experimental strategies. Lancet Neurol 2014;13:1241–1256
25. Caggiano AO, Zimber MP, Ganguly A, Blight AR, Gruskin EA. Chondroitinase ABCI improves locomotion and bladder function following contusion injury of the rat spinal cord. J Neurotrauma 2005;22:226–239
26. Bartus K, James ND, Didangelos A, et al. Large-scale chondroitin sulfate proteoglycan digestion with chondroitinase gene therapy leads to reduced pathology and modulates macrophage phenotype following spinal cord contusion injury. J Neurosci 2014;34:4822–4836
27. Lee YS, Lin CY, Jiang HH, Depaul M, Lin VW, Silver J. Nerve regeneration restores supraspinal control of bladder function after complete spinal cord injury. J Neurosci 2013;33:10591–10606
28. Lee H, McKeon RJ, Bellamkonda RV. Sustained delivery of thermostabilized chABC enhances axonal sprouting and functional recovery after spinal cord injury. Proc Natl Acad Sci U S A 2010;107:3340–3345
29. James ND, Shea J, Muir EM, Verhaagen J, Schneider BL, Bradbury EJ. Chondroitinase gene therapy improves upper limb function following cervical contusion injury. Exp Neurol 2015;271:131–135

30. Yoo M, Khaled M, Gibbs KM, et al. Arylsulfatase B improves locomotor function after mouse spinal cord injury. PLoS ONE 2013;8:e57415

31. Smith JS, Anderson R, Pham T, Bhatia N, Steward O, Gupta R. Role of early surgical decompression of the intradural space after cervical spinal cord injury in an animal model. J Bone Joint Surg Am 2010;92:1206–1214

32. Klapka N, Hermanns S, Straten G, et al. Suppression of fibrous scarring in spinal cord injury of rat promotes long-distance regeneration of corticospinal tract axons, rescue of primary motoneurons in somatosensory cortex and significant functional recovery. Eur J Neurosci 2005;22:3047–3058

33. Norenberg MD, Smith J, Marcillo A. The pathology of human spinal cord injury: defining the problems. J Neurotrauma 2004;21:429–440

34. Logan A, Baird A, Berry M. Decorin attenuates gliotic scar formation in the rat cerebral hemisphere. Exp Neurol 1999;159:504–510

35. Davies JE, Tang X, Denning JW, Archibald SJ, Davies SJA. Decorin suppresses neurocan, brev ican, phosphacan and NG2 expression and promotes axon growth across adult rat spinal cord injuries. Eur J Neurosci 2004;19:1226–1242

36. Oudega M, Chao OY, Avison DL, et al. Systemic administration of a deoxyribozyme to xylosyltransferase-1 mRNA promotes recovery after a spinal cord contusion injury. Exp Neurol 2012;237:170–179

37. McKillop WM, Dragan M, Schedl A, Brown A. Conditional Sox9 ablation reduces chondroitin sulfate proteoglycan levels and improves motor function following spinal cord injury. Glia 2013;61:164–177

38. Takeuchi K, Yoshioka N, Higa Onaga S, et al. Chondroitin sulphate N-acetylgalactosaminyl-transferase-1 inhibits recovery from neural injury. Nat Commun 2013;4:2740

39. Maier IC, Ichiyama RM, Courtine G, et al. Differential effects of anti-Nogo-A antibody treatment and treadmill training in rats with incomplete spinal cord injury. Brain 2009;132(Pt 6):1426–1440

40. Marsh BC, Astill SL, Utley A, Ichiyama RM. Movement rehabilitation after spinal cord injuries: emerging concepts and future directions. Brain Res Bull 2011;84:327–336

41. Girgis J, Merrett D, Kirkland S, Metz GAS, Verge V, Fouad K. Reaching training in rats with spinal cord injury promotes plasticity and task specific recovery. Brain 2007;130(Pt 11):2993–3003

42. García-Alías G, Barkhuysen S, Buckle M, Fawcett JW. Chondroitinase ABC treatment opens a window of opportunity for task-specific rehabilitation. Nat Neurosci 2009;12:1145–1151

43. Wang D, Ichiyama RM, Zhao R, Andrews MR, Fawcett JW. Chondroitinase combined with rehabilitation promotes recovery of forelimb function in rats with chronic spinal cord injury. J Neurosci 2011;31:9332–9344

12

Functional Electrical Stimulation and Neuromodulation Approaches to Enhance Recovery After Spinal Cord Injury

César Márquez-Chin, Emilie Sagripanti, and Milos R. Popovic

▤ Introduction

Spinal cord injury (SCI) can result in total or partial loss of the ability to perform voluntary movements and to experience somatosensory sensations. The injury disrupts the natural communication between the brain and the peripheral nervous system, making it difficult or impossible for both efferent and afferent signals to act on their intended targets. The lost motor and/or sensory function typically occurs below the level of injury, so that a high level of lesion in the spinal cord (e.g., at the level of the cervical vertebrae) may result in the lower limbs, trunk, and upper limbs being affected, whereas a lesion at the thoracic level may result in impaired function of the trunk and lower limbs only. Some of the functions that may be affected by SCI include walking, sitting, grasping, bladder voiding, and blood pressure regulation. In addition to the level of injury, the severity of the impairment can also be influenced by whether the spinal cord has been severed completely or incompletely, which results in complete or partial function loss, respectively.

Improvements in acute and subacute care of SCI has resulted in an increased number of patients who are able to recover function to varying degrees, depending on the nature of the injury and other health variables. This has changed the way we view rehabilitation for this population, and has coincided with emerging technologies that can be applied to facilitate the rehabilitation process.

The limitations resulting from the decreased motor and sensory function can have catastrophic effects on the individuals who have sustained an SCI and on their families. As a consequence, great efforts are being applied to developing knowledge and technology to mitigate or eliminate the effects of SCI. This chapter discusses the use of functional electrical stimulation (FES) as a method of restoring voluntary function after paralysis.

▤ Functional Electrical Stimulation

Using Electrical Stimulation to Produce Movement

The production of muscle contractions using electrical stimulation is possible due to the excitability nature of nerve cells. A brief change in the potential of the nerve cell membrane from $-80/-90$ mV to $-40/-50$ mV, in response to electrical stimulation, is sufficient to generate an action potential. Action potentials are the main mechanism by which information is transmitted in the nervous system. For example, in some cases the rate at which action potentials are generated is proportional to the intensity of a stimulus. They are the result of a sequence of events involving movement of different molecules across the cellular membrane through specific cell structures, some of which respond to electrical changes. This makes it possible to use electrical discharges to generate action potentials artificially by forcing a change in the electric potential across a nerve cell membrane.

The therapeutic use of electrical stimulation has progressed significantly over the past 50 years. Initially, neuromuscular electrical stimulation (NMES) was applied to weak muscles to improve strength and endurance, and occasionally, with limited success, to reduce spasticity. It soon became evident that this modality worked best when the patient was actively engaged in producing the movements that the NMES was assisting. NMES later evolved into FES, in which the technology was applied to work as an assistive device, often called a *neuroprosthesis*, which the patient wears daily during functional activities or has it implanted in the body.

Neuroprosthesis

A neuroprosthesis is a device that produces motor and/or sensory functions by applying short bursts of electrical impulses to the central or peripheral nervous system. The resulting action potentials in muscles and nerve cells can be used clinically to compensate for abnormal or absent neurologic function. Neuroprostheses serve many purposes and therefore come in different forms. They can be used, for example, to stimulate the basal ganglia to eliminate tremor in patients with Parkinson's disease, or to aid in the perception of sound by stimulating the auditory nerve of the cochlea. In this chapter, we use the term *neuroprosthesis* to refer to technology that restores voluntary motor function through electrical stimulation.

What Is Functional Electrical Stimulation?

By applying carefully controlled stimulation sequences to innervated muscles, it is possible to achieve complex synergistic movements such as reaching, grasping, and walking. This type of neuroprosthesis is often referred to as FES, as it produces functional and coordinated movements. FES systems are envisioned as devices for patients with upper motor neuron disorders such as stroke, SCI, or traumatic brain injury. In these populations, the devices are used to artificially produce the movement that patients are unable to carry out independently.

Delivery of FES can be controlled using simple manual devices such as switches, dials, and sliders, all of which can be mounted on assistive devices including a cane, a walker, or a wheelchair. The electrical stimulation can be delivered using surface (transcutaneous), percutaneous, or implanted electrodes, which have advantages and disadvantages that make them more suitable for specific applications, as described in the following subsections.

Surface Electrodes

Surface electrodes, which are applied to the skin, are noninvasive, easy to apply, and generally inexpensive. Typical magnitudes of the electrical currents used with these electrodes range between 5 and 120 mA, which is greater than the intensity required when applying stimulation using percutaneous or implanted electrodes. Although highly versatile and suitable for temporary use, surface electrodes are often incapable of stimulating deep muscles (e.g., hip flexors) without producing unintended contractions in other neighboring muscles. This can be partially avoided by using arrays of electrodes with several electrical contacts to increase selectivity.

Percutaneous Electrodes

Percutaneous electrodes are thin wires that are inserted through the skin into muscular tissue. These remain in place temporarily and are used only for short-term FES interventions, although there are cases in the literature where certain individuals had the electrodes implanted for months and even years. The current amplitudes used with percutaneous stimulation rarely exceed 25 mA. As with implanted electrodes, local infection is possible.

Implanted Electrodes

Implanted electrodes are permanently inserted, have higher stimulation selectivity, and require the lowest stimulation intensity, both desirable aspects for FES systems. However, their application requires invasive surgery, which always carries a risk of infection. The current amplitudes used with implanted stimulation also rarely exceed 25 mA.

Applications of Functional Electrical Stimulation

There are two main applications of FES technology. First, it can be used as an orthotic/neuroprosthetic device worn every day (or implanted in the body) to increase independence in activities of daily living by facilitating movement that would otherwise be impossible due to paralysis. Second, it can be used temporarily as a form of short-term therapy to help the neuromuscular system relearn functions impaired due to an insult to the nervous system. This latter approach is intended to promote recovery of voluntary function, and the use of FES is discontinued after the therapy is completed. This application was developed after users of NMES and FES systems reported improvements in their motor function to the point that they did not require the neuroprosthesis any longer.

The next sections provide examples of both applications in the context of restoration of movement after SCI.

Functional Electrical Stimulation Applications as an Orthotic/Neuroprosthetic Device

Neuroprostheses for Standing

Functional electrical stimulation can be used to facilitate standing, a function that is often impaired after SCI. This is achieved by regulating the movements of the ankle joints using FES. To assist with trunk control, it is possible to use additional devices such as standing frames, full-body orthoses, or electrical stimulation as well. The FES-assisted standing has been demonstrated primarily in individuals with an SCI at the thoracic level, but the complexity of the required setups (e.g., full body casting and support frames) used in such experiments often make this technology unsuitable for clinical use at the present time.

One important example is the Case Western Reserve University/Department of Veterans Affairs (CWRU-VA) standing neuroprosthesis, which creates an upright posture by activating the muscles of the trunk, hips, and thigh bilaterally using an 8- to 16-channel implanted stimulator. With the addition of an orthosis the CWRU-VA enables the user to achieve more than 10 minute of uninterrupted upright stance.[1] However, this system does not provide balance control, so the user has to rely on a walker or a similar device to ensure balance during standing. In addition, this device uses an open-loop control scheme, which results in quicker muscular fatigue.

Neuroprostheses for Walking

Kralj and colleagues[2] created an FES system for walking that integrated reflex action in its design. In this approach, surface electrodes are placed over the quadriceps muscles and peroneal nerves on both legs. The users can activate the stimulation using external buttons placed

SCI in an intervention lasting 12 to 18 weeks.[4] Walking was produced by stimulating the muscles directly instead of activation of the flexor withdrawal reflex (as described above[2]). Participants showed improved walking speed, stride length, and stepping frequency, among other improvements.

Encouraged by the findings reported by Thrasher et al,[4] our team performed the first-ever phase II randomized controlled trial in chronic (≥ 18 months), traumatic, incomplete [American Spinal Injury Association (ASIA) Impairment Scale (AIS) grades C and D], C2 to T12 SCI individuals.[5] The FEST protocol and the stimulator used in this study was identical to the one used by Thrasher et al. The study clearly demonstrated that FEST for walking was able to improve locomotion function in the selected patient population and to generate clinically meaningful improvements, with significantly better outcomes on the Spinal Cord Independence Measure Mobility subscore following FEST compared with non-FES exercise intervention.

Functional Electrical Stimulation Therapy for Improving Upper Limb Function

Partial or complete loss of grasping and reaching functions may result from SCI at T1 level or above. Over the years various teams that have investigated the use of FEST for grasping in the SCI population have shown that this therapy has an ability to improve upper limb function. Popović et al[12] demonstrated the efficacy of the Bionic Glove to improve upper limb function in individuals with C5–C7 SCI, which was the first concrete evidence that FEST can improve grasping. In addition, using the ETHZ-Para Care (ETH Zurich, Zurich) grasping neuroprosthesis, originally used as an orthosis, Mangold et al[16] demonstrated that a few patients with SCI experienced a weak carryover effect (i.e., FEST effect) following intensive training with the neuroprosthesis for grasping.

Our team has also observed the positive impact that FEST has on the grasping function of individuals with SCI at C3–C7 with impaired motor function (AIS grades A, B, C, and D). We recently completed a randomized controlled trial with 21 participants with incomplete SCI at the C3–C7 levels during the first 6 months after their injury (subacute).[17] The subjects received 40 therapy sessions of 1-hour duration, 5 days a week for 8 weeks, to improve their upper limb function. They were randomized into an intervention group (FEST) or a control group. The intervention group received 1 hour of conventional occupational therapy followed by 1 hour of FEST. The control group received 2 hours of conventional occupational therapy. The intervention group showed significantly larger improvements in upper limb function as measured by the Spinal Cord Independence Measure Self-Care subscore. In addition, the participants who received FEST for grasping increased or maintained these functional gains 6 months after the therapy was completed.

Our team also performed a pilot randomized controlled trial to examine if the FEST could be used to improve voluntary grasping function in individuals with chronic (≥ 24 months), incomplete (AIS grades B–D), C4 to C7 SCI. Although only eight individuals participated in the study, the results clearly suggest that 39 hours of FEST for grasping in this patient population is more effective than an equivalent amount of conventional occupation therapy.

Since its launch on the Canadian market, therapists have used MyndMove to deliver FEST in the SCI population, not only for grasping (the above studies investigated FEST for grasping only) but also for reaching. The preliminary and unofficial reports suggest that FEST can be used with individuals with chronic and subacute SCI to improve both reaching and grasping functions, and that future studies are needed to investigate the efficiency of FEST for both reaching and grasping in the SCI population.

Potential Mechanisms of Recovery in Functional Electrical Stimulation Therapy

The mechanisms by which FEST produces recovery of voluntary function are unknown. However, there are physical and neurologic aspects that may explain the effects of this therapeutic intervention. Three possible peripheral mechanisms can be considered. First, simply by muscle training and strengthening, FEST may improve residual muscle function. Second, FEST may increase the flexibility and range of motion in the affected limb, improving voluntary function as well. Third, FEST may reduce muscle spasticity, resulting in improved motor function, although there is conflicting evidence on this effect.

From a neurologic perspective, improvements due to FEST may be explained through cortical reorganization, which has been found after injury to the central nervous system (CNS). One potential mechanism stems from the fact that FES is likely to activate both motor and sensory nerve fibers, which, combined with the forced repetitive movements used in FEST, may promote neuroplastic changes in the CNS. Also, task-specific training rehabilitation has been shown to produce greater cortical reorganization and plasticity compared with traditional therapy. With these factors in mind, using repetitive FES movements that provide sensory stimulation can likely promote neuroplasticity in the CNS.[18]

Rushton[19] suggested that the orthodromic and antidromic impulses generated when a nerve fiber is stimulated with FES may result in reorganization beyond the cerebral cortex, resulting in the FES carryover effect. During FES, a voluntary command descending from the brain to a spinal motor neuron can meet the antidromic impulse at the motor neuron. These two impulses at the spinal cord can strengthen the synaptic connection via Hebb's rule, leading to increased efficacy of the voluntary descending command to activate the impaired muscle in individuals with SCI.

A final potential explanation that supports the mechanisms behind FEST, proposed by Popovic et al,[17] includes the incorporation of sensory feedback. If FEST is used to assist in performing a motor task while voluntarily generating the corresponding motor command (i.e., attempting the movement), FEST provides afferent feedback confirming that the desired command was executed successfully. The repetitive combination of the corresponding efferent and afferent signals in the CNS, for prolonged periods of time, may facilitate functional reorganization and retraining of unaffected and functionally related areas of the CNS, enabling the functional parts of the CNS to take control over the damaged parts to improve outcomes following FEST. The combination of the motor task repetition, diverse and meaningful tasks, and the individual's full engagement and attention to the tasks performed (all three being hallmarks of FEST) plays a critical role in retraining voluntary motor function.

The carryover effect of FEST needs to be fully examined and explained, as it is most likely multifactorial. However, it is certain that FEST is very effective at restoring voluntary functions in individuals following SCI. As for FEST for locomotion, we have indications that it is able to restore voluntary walking in individuals after SCI. However, it is our impression that the FEST for walking may require further refinement and clinical trials before it will be able to achieve the same robust outcomes as FEST for reaching and gasping.

Potential Future Directions for Functional Electrical Stimulation Therapy

The FES technology, used either as an assistive device or as a tool to enhance voluntary function, continues to evolve. New electrode shapes and configurations, stimulation sequences, and techniques are among the things that are shaping the next generation of neuroprosthetic technology. One of the most exciting developments in the field of FEST is its intersection with brain–computer interfacing (BCI) technology. A BCI translates brain signals into control commands for external devices such as computers, augmentative and alternative communication devices, and robotic systems. Operation of BCIs does not require any voluntary movement (e.g., to activate a switch), which positions BCI systems as a potentially enormous opportunity to assist individuals whose ability to move voluntarily is very limited or nonexistent.

A BCI analyzes the activity of the brain to extract properties reflective of a person's intent. These attributes may include evoked potentials, power of specific frequency bands, and the frequency of firing of individual neurons. The features are then transformed into commands specific to the device to be controlled.

Virtually any method to monitor the activity of the brain can be used to implement these brain interfaces. Magnetoencephalography (MEG), functional magnetic resonance imaging (fMRI), and near-infrared spectroscopy (NIRS) have all been used to create BCI technology. However, most BCIs are implemented using electrical recordings of the brain. These include intracortical recordings, electrocorticography (ECoG), and electroencephalography (EEG). To date, most BCI systems have been created using EEG techniques, likely due to their noninvasive nature, relative low cost, widespread availability, speed, and rich information content that they provide.

One important approach, widely used for implementing EEG-based BCI systems, consists of transforming the power changes of sensorimotor rhythms into a control signal. This is due to the fact that it is possible to learn to produce changes in amplitude within the α (8 to 12 Hz) and β (13 to 30 Hz) frequency ranges by imagining movements.[20] These changes are present in ECoG signals too, which also display changes at higher frequencies not typically associated with EEG. Uses for this technology have included computer cursor control as well as wheelchair driving and ambulation in a virtual reality environment, among others. In addition, and perhaps due to the fact that activation of the BCI is achieved through imagination of movements, applications have also focused on the control of orthotic and prosthetic devices designed to facilitate voluntary function of paralyzed or missing limbs. More specifically, individuals with SCI have controlled a hand orthosis,[21] a noninvasive[14,22] and implanted neuroprosthesis for grasping,[23] and, more recently, a neuroprosthesis for walking.[24]

Brain–Computer Interfacing Technology for Neurorehabilitation

Similar to FES technology, BCI technology has experienced a shift in its conceived application. One of the original intended uses of BCI technology was to provide a means of communication for individuals with locked-in syndrome who are completely unable to communicate due to a complete loss of the ability to move voluntarily. Patients with advanced amyotrophic lateral sclerosis (ALS) and brainstem stroke were the populations targeted by early BCI systems. However, in the last decade, there has been great interest in the use of BCI technology as a tool to promote recovery of voluntary function after stroke and SCI.

It is likely that at the core of this interest lies the fact that the use of BCI technology, and particularly when its operation requires users to imagine that they are moving a part of their bodies (e.g., a hand or a foot), overlaps factors that have been identified as important to facilitate changes in the nervous system that can lead to motor recovery.[25] For example, operation of a BCI requires full attention for its operation (e.g., focus on the imagined movement). Focus on the movement being practiced during therapy is also important. In FEST, this is achieved by asking patients to attempt the practiced movement and by triggering the stimulation only after a few seconds of effort. In addition, the use of a BCI engages the CNS directly, without applying electrical of magnetic fields to the brain, and without focusing exclusively on peripheral activity (i.e., limb movement). At the moment, the reports describing the use of a BCI for rehabilitation of voluntary movement are restricted to patients with stroke excluding the SCI population. However, the principles behind using a BCI for rehabilitation after stroke may be applicable to patients with SCI as well.

Brain–Computer Interfacing Technology as a Short-Term Rehabilitation Tool

An Addition to Therapy

At the moment, there are two main approaches to integrate BCI technology into the rehabilitation of individuals with limited mobility. The first one consists of using the BCI as a tool to enable patients to learn to produce normal oscillatory activity as related to voluntary movement (i.e., changes in power in the α and β frequency ranges produced by motor imagery). This intervention is motivated by the hypothesis that the changes in the nervous system responsible for producing normal brain activity will result in increased normal function of the nervous system, leading to improved motor control. Interventions using this approach have included BCI as an addition to regular physical therapy.

In a recent study, Ramos-Murguialday et al[26] reported increased recovery of voluntary arm and hand function in 32 chronic stroke patients who used a motor-imagery–based BCI immediately before their regular physical therapy sessions. Participants in the experimental group underwent training sessions to produce voluntary power decreases in sensorimotor rhythms to control hand and arm orthoses, whereas activation of these devices was random for the control group. The activity of the brain was recorded using EEG electrodes placed over the ipsilesional motor cortex. Both groups received physiotherapy immediately after using the BCI. The experimental group showed significant increases in upper limb function at the end of the intervention, which were not observed for the control group.

Brain–Computer Interfacing to Control Movement Facilitation Technologies

The second approach for integrating BCI into rehabilitation consists of detecting the patient's intention to move and trigger an external device to facilitate the intended movement. The motivation behind this intervention is that the artificially produced movement will generate sensory feedback that, combined with the intention to move, will produce changes in the CNS, resulting in improved motor function. One of the most widely explored interventions to date using this approach has been the triggering of robotic rehabilitation systems. For example, Ang et al[27] conducted a randomized controlled trial in which patients with stroke underwent upper limb therapy using a robotic system to facilitate two-dimensional reaching movements. Both the experimental and control groups were instructed to reach to eight different targets placed radially, and in both cases the robot provided assistance to complete the movement. Triggering of the robot was done automatically or using mechanical cues (control group), or using a BCI operated by motor imagery (experimental group). Their results demonstrated a significant and comparable increase in arm function after 4 weeks of treatment for both groups, with the experimental group achieving these results with much lower intensity therapy (136 repetitions per session and 1,040 repetitions per session for the experimental and control groups, respectively).

Delivery of FEST triggered by a BCI is in its infancy (**Fig. 12.3**). Thus, there is little reported work, with much of it still at a stage of feasibility testing. Combining FES with a BCI poses significant technical problems, as the stimulation used to produce movement can generate interference affecting the reliability of measuring EEG signals. However, the possibility that the rich proprioceptive and somatosensory feedback produced by the electrical stimulation, coupled with a verified intention to perform a motor task, makes the integration of FEST and

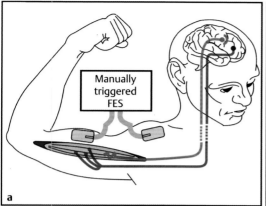
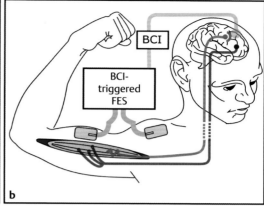

Fig. 12.3 Functional electrical stimulation (FES) therapy and brain–computer interface (BCI) integration. These conceptual illustrations depict possible configurations for integrating a neuroprosthesis for motor restoration and a BCI in the context of FES therapy. **(a)** Current FES therapy relies on a therapist to identify the patient's intention to move and trigger the stimulation after a few seconds. The motor command is met with corresponding sensory information, which may play a role in the restoration of function observed after FES therapy. **(b)** A BCI-triggered FES system would identify the patient's intention to move through motor-related changes in electroencephalography (EEG) activity. This would ensure that the patient is engaged and focused in the task, and that the stimulation is delivered immediately when the movement is attempted. (Courtesy of REL.)

BCI technology very promising for restoring voluntary movement after stroke and SCI (**Figs. 12.3** and **12.4**).

In one important study, Daly et al[25] explored the efficacy of BCI-controlled FEST to restore voluntary finger function 10 months after stroke in a single subject, a woman who had lost the ability to move her fingers individually. She was asked to attempt movements with her index finger. A BCI detected her intention to move, reflected as a decrease of power in the β frequency range, which triggered an FES system to facilitate the finger movement. After nine sessions, the participant's ability to perform finger extension increased. Our group also examined the use of BCI systems combined with FEST for grasping in able-bodied individuals. In that work, we were interested in the neuroplastic changes induced in the motor cortex by such a system immediately following the therapy as compared with FEST alone.[28] This pilot study demonstrated that a BCI-driven FEST system for grasping is more effective in inducing neuroplasticity in able-bodied individuals as compared with conventional FEST system.

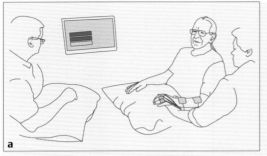
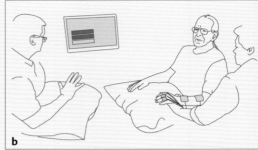
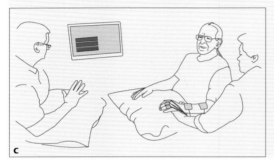
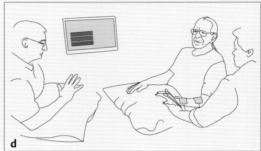

Fig. 12.4 Brain–computer interface (BCI)-triggered neuroprosthesis for grasping for FES therapy. The images illustrate the operation of a prototype BCI-controlled neuroprosthesis for its use in FES therapy to restore upper limb function. The system, which used a single EEG electrode, was tested with a 64-year-old man who had a stroke 6 years earlier, resulting in severe hemiplegia. **(a)** The patient was asked to relax and prepare to open his hand. **(b)** An experimenter demonstrates the movement to perform, which also serves as a cue for the patient to attempt the movement. **(c)** The BCI detects the intention to move (the change in color of the bottom square box on the screen, from white **(b)** to green **(c)** indicates a change in the BCI user interface). **(d)** The BCI triggers the stimulation opening the patient's hand. The sequence of events was completed in 4 seconds. (Courtesy of REL.)

■ Conclusion

Functional electrical stimulation has been successful as a method to improve function after SCI. Whether used as an orthotic system daily to produce the movement impossible to carry out voluntarily after SCI, or as a short-term therapeutic intervention to promote recovery of voluntary function, FES technology can have a direct positive impact on the quality of life of individuals with SCI. It is, however, a technology that continues to evolve in both its engineering and its applications. As we see important advances in the field of BCI, it is likely that integration of these two technologies (FES and BCI) will become an important addition to the tools available for restoring motor function.

■ Chapter Summary

Functional electrical stimulation, which delivers highly controlled low-energy electrical discharges to produce contractions in paralyzed muscles, can be used to restore movements, including standing, walking, reaching, and grasping. In addition, when used temporarily as a therapeutic intervention, this technology has produced some remarkable recoveries of voluntary motor function. This chapter described the technology and its applications to restore voluntary movement after an SCI. We also described the integration of functional electrical stimulation technology with brain–computer interfaces as a potential next step in the evolution of this field.

Pearls

- Functional electrical stimulation (FES) can produce functional and complex movements by applying highly controlled low-voltage electrical impulses to paralyzed muscles.
- FES technology can be used as a permanent orthotic device or as part of a short-term rehabilitation program.
- FES therapy uses FES technology as a temporary therapeutic intervention to promote neuroplasticity and produce clinically meaningful and long-lasting recovery of voluntary movement after spinal cord injury.
- Improvements in voluntary function after FES therapy apply to both complete and incomplete SCI, and both subacute and chronic patients benefited from this therapy.

Pitfalls

- The contemporary FES therapy produces contractions only in innervated muscles, that is, muscles whose peripheral nerves are intact.
- The complexity of some FES systems confines them to clinical and research environments.
- Muscle deconditioning, muscle fatigue, contractures, inability to selectively activate targeted muscles, and discomfort during stimulation are common obstacles in delivering FES therapy. However, advanced FES systems have been able to overcome these and other similar challenges.
- It is common to change stimulation protocols multiple times during a single FES therapy session to facilitate different movements. This requires repositioning of the stimulation electrodes, which reduces the active therapy time.

References

Five Must-Read References

1. Kobetic R, Triolo RJ, Uhlir JP, et al. Implanted functional electrical stimulation system for mobility in paraplegia: a follow-up case report. IEEE Trans Rehabil Eng 1999;7:390–398
2. Kralj A, Bajd T, Turk R. Enhancement of gait restoration in spinal injured patients by functional electrical stimulation. Clin Orthop Relat Res 1988;233:34–43
3. Andrews BJ, Baxendale RH, Barnett R, Phillips GF, Yamazaki T, Paul JP, Freeman PA. Hybrid FES orthosis incorporating closed loop control and sensory feedback. J Biomed Eng, 1988;10(2)189–195.
4. Thrasher TA, Flett HM, Popovic MR. Gait training regimen for incomplete spinal cord injury using functional electrical stimulation. Spinal Cord 2006;44:357–361
5. Kapadia N, Masani K, Catharine Craven B, et al. A randomized trial of functional electrical stimulation for walking in incomplete spinal cord injury: effects on walking competency. J Spinal Cord Med 2014;37:511–524
6. Dimitrijevic MR, Gerasimenko Y, Pinter MM. Evidence for a spinal central pattern generator in humans. Ann N Y Acad Sci 1998;860:360–376
7. Harkema S, Gerasimenko Y, Hodes J, et al. Effect of epidural stimulation of the lumbosacral spinal cord on voluntary movement, standing, and assisted stepping after motor complete paraplegia: a case study. Lancet 2011;377:1938–1947

8. Angeli CA, Edgerton VR, Gerasimenko YP, Harkema SJ. Altering spinal cord excitability enables voluntary movements after chronic complete paralysis in humans. Brain 2014;137(Pt 5):1394–1409
9. Smith B, Tang Z, Johnson MW, et al. An externally powered, multichannel, implantable stimulator-telemeter for control of paralyzed muscle. IEEE Trans Biomed Eng 1998;45:463–475
10. Hendricks HT, IJzerman MJ, de Kroon JR, in 't Groen FA, Zilvold G. Functional electrical stimulation by means of the "Ness Handmaster Orthosis" in chronic stroke patients: an exploratory study. Clin Rehabil 2001;15:217–220
11. Prochazka A, Gauthier M, Wieler M, Kenwell Z. The bionic glove: an electrical stimulator garment that provides controlled grasp and hand opening in quadriplegia. Arch Phys Med Rehabil 1997;78:608–614
12. Popović D, Stojanović A, Pjanović A, et al. Clinical evaluation of the bionic glove. Arch Phys Med Rehabil 1999;80:299–304
13. Popovic MR, Keller T. Modular transcutaneous functional electrical stimulation system. Med Eng Phys 2005;27:81–92
14. Márquez-Chin C, Popovic MR, Cameron T, Lozano AM, Chen R. Control of a neuroprosthesis for grasping using off-line classification of electrocorticographic signals: case study. Spinal Cord 2009;47:802–808
15. Bajd T, Kralj A, Stefancic M, Lavrac N. Use of functional electrical stimulation in the lower extremities

of incomplete spinal cord injured patients. Artif Organs 1999;23:403–409

16. Mangold S, Keller T, Curt A, Dietz V. Transcutaneous functional electrical stimulation for grasping in subjects with .cervical spinal cord injury. Spinal Cord 2005;43:1–13

17. Popovic MR, Kapadia N, Zivanovic V, Furlan JC, Craven BC, McGillivray C. Functional electrical stimulation therapy of voluntary grasping versus only conventional rehabilitation for patients with subacute incomplete tetraplegia: a randomized clinical trial. Neurorehabil Neural Repair 2011;25:433–442

18. Bigland-Ritchie B, Kukulka CG, Lippold OC, Woods JJ. The absence of neuromuscular transmission failure in sustained maximal voluntary contractions. J Physiol 1982;330:265–278

19. Rushton DN. Functional electrical stimulation and rehabilitation—an hypothesis. Med Eng Phys 2003; 25:75–78

20. Pfurtscheller G, Flotzinger D, Kalcher J. Brain-computer interface—a new communication device for handicapped persons. Journal of Microcomputer Applications. 1993;16:293–299

21. Pfurtscheller G, Guger C, Müller G, Krausz G, Neuper C. Brain oscillations control hand orthosis in a tetraplegic. Neurosci Lett 2000;292:211–214

22. Pfurtscheller G, Müller GR, Pfurtscheller J, Gerner HJ, Rupp R. "Thought"-control of functional electrical stimulation to restore hand grasp in a patient with tetraplegia. Neurosci Lett 2003;351:33–36

23. Müller-Putz GR, Scherer R, Pfurtscheller G, Rupp R. EEG-based neuroprosthesis control: a step towards clinical practice. Neurosci Lett 2005;382:169–174

24. King CE, Wang PT, McCrimmon CM, Chou CC, Do AH, Nenadic Z. The feasibility of a brain-computer interface functional electrical stimulation system for the restoration of overground walking after paraplegia. J Neuroeng Rehabil 2015;12:80

25. Daly JJ, Cheng R, Rogers J, Litinas K, Hrovat K, Dohring M. Feasibility of a new application of noninvasive Brain Computer Interface (BCI): a case study of training for recovery of volitional motor control after stroke. J Neurol Phys Ther 2009;33:203–211

26. Ramos-Murguialday A, Broetz D, Rea M, et al. Brain-machine interface in chronic stroke rehabilitation: a controlled study. Ann Neurol 2013;74:100–108

27. Ang KK, Chua KSG, Phua KS, et al. A randomized controlled trial of EEG-based motor imagery brain-computer interface robotic rehabilitation for stroke. Clin EEG Neurosci 2014

28. McGie SC, Zariffa J, Popovic MR, Nagai MK. Short-term neuroplastic effects of brain-controlled and muscle-controlled electrical stimulation. Neuromodulation 2014

Advanced Rehabilitation Strategies for Individuals with Traumatic Spinal Cord Injury

William Z. Rymer, Sheila Burt, and Arun Jayaraman

▤ Introduction

Traumatic spinal cord injury (SCI) can severely impact a person's upper and lower limb motor function. Consequently, many patients with SCI list the ability to regain some walking movement and arm/hand strength as top priorities.[1] Although emergency care and early therapeutic programs for persons with SCI have dramatically improved in recent decades, enormous physical barriers are still faced by patients and clinicians in establishing safe standing and walking therapies, as well as therapies that help restore upper limb strength and function. A substantial body of literature drawn from experiments on animal models has shown that imposing locomotor movements in animals with incomplete SCI can help to retrain dormant spinal neural circuits and enable these circuits to generate relatively normal oscillatory neural activation patterns during recovery.[2] These animal data have been interpreted as supporting the analogous idea that retraining human locomotor function after SCI by externally imposing near-normal movement patterns on the lower extremities may have similar beneficial effects. This type of therapy entails externally imposing cyclical leg movements on patients recovering locomotor function while safely supporting them. These technologies may also reduce the prevalence of secondary medical conditions associated with SCI.[3] However, many of these training strategies, such as body weight–supported treadmill training, are labor-intensive endeavors that require the time and effort of several physical therapists to assist with proper loading of the limbs and weight transfers.

This reality has stimulated a burgeoning interest in the development of advanced engineering and robotic technologies to assist and augment therapist actions in patients with SCI. However, developing safe, low-cost, and clinically effective devices constitutes a major physical and engineering challenge. Robotic devices have also been developed to provide assistance or therapy for the impaired upper limb, although the scientific basis for improving upper limb function through movement training is more limited. This chapter focuses on the characteristics and impact of several robotic devices that are currently available, reviews the current research findings with the most prevalent versions, and discusses the value of emerging wearable sensor systems for monitoring training efficacy of advanced technologies.

Treadmill-Based Robotic Devices

Rehabilitation strategies for individuals with SCI focus on those with incomplete SCI, and use task-specific repetitive training to increase neural drive to the lower limbs, strengthen leg muscles, and potentially restore some degree of useful limb function. It is widely believed that intensive task-specific practice promotes the emergence of neural plasticity, which is mediated by structural and functional changes in neural circuits. In the past 30 years, several robotic trainers have been developed that can augment and sometimes replace the physical actions of therapists to help restore upper- or lower-limb function, and improve a patient's gait, balance, and posture.

Providing body-weight support through a harness may enable patients to begin therapy earlier in recovery, despite weakness or poor coordination, and remove the risk and fear of falling. In the following subsections we review some robotic trainers for the upper and lower limb.

The Lokomat

The Lokomat (Hocoma Inc., Norwell, MA, and Volketswil, Switzerland), one of the most studied robotic gait training systems and the most widely adopted, was developed as the outcome of a collaboration between Hocoma and researchers at Balgrist University Hospital in Zurich.[4] An initial prototype was developed in 1999. There are now two versions of the machine: the Lokomat®Pro (**Fig. 13.1**) and the Lokomat®Nanos. The Nanos was launched in 2010, and offered a smaller version of the Lokomat®Pro for rooms with a ceiling height of at least 240 cm (~ 7.9 feet). The Lokomat is an exoskeleton, mounted above a treadmill, with extensive body-weight support technologies

included. The device uses linear actuators to control joint angles at the knee and hip. In older models, movements were externally imposed in the form of a predetermined normal gait pattern, irrespective of movement generated by the user, and were limited to the sagittal plane. These constraints limited the opportunity for balance training and did not require users to generate voluntary movements on their own. A new optional module, "FreeD," supports weight shifts and promotes balance recovery through lateral and rotational movements of the pelvis. Software provides game-like exercises that are used to motivate patients. To induce greater efforts, the movements are scored to encourage patients to make correct physical actions. Software provides game-like exercises that are used to motivate patients and induce greater effort, and movements are scored to encourage patients to make correct movements.

Individuals with incomplete SCI (American Spinal Injury Association [ASIA] grades C and D) showed significant improvements in overground gait speed and endurance after 12 weeks of training on earlier versions of the Lokomat,[5] although this did not translate into improved functional walking ability. Generally, individuals with the most impaired locomotor and functional abilities showed the greatest improvements after training. Therefore, the device developers recommend its use preferentially for nonambulatory persons with incomplete SCI. In a small study, three individuals with incomplete SCI also demonstrated improved gait speed, endurance, and ASIA scores after 16 to 20 weeks of training.[6] A study involving 60 patients with incomplete SCI in which Lokomat training in addition to traditional over-ground training was compared with over-ground training alone found that robot-assisted training may have increased benefit over conventional training alone.[7]

The Aretech ZeroG

The Aretech ZeroG® (Aretech LLC, Ashburn, VA) is a robotic gait and balance training system designed to enable patients with a variety of

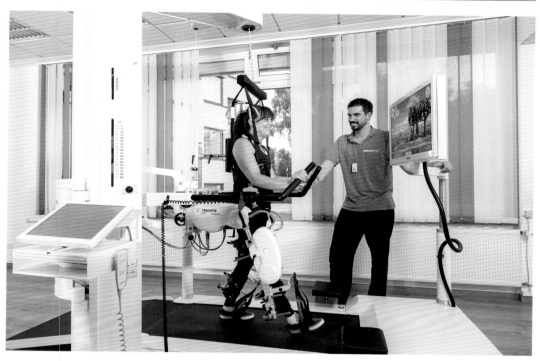

Fig. 13.1 The Lokomat was developed in collaboration by Hocoma and researchers at Balgrist University Hospital in Zurich. It is one of the most studied robotic gait training systems and the most widely adopted. (Courtesy of Hocoma, Volketswil, Switzerland.)

neurologic impairments to practice walking, balancing, and performing other functional activities while supported by an overhead harness, suspended from a ceiling-mounted track.[8] There are three versions of the device: ZeroG, which provides over-ground bodyweight or balance/static support; ZeroG Lite, which provides treadmill-based support; and ZeroG Passive, which is a fall protection system. This discussion focuses on the ZeroG for bodyweight support training (referred to simply as the ZeroG; **Fig. 13.2**). Developed with United States Military funding by Joe Hidler, PhD, at the National Rehabilitation Hospital, Washington, DC, and a team of engineers and therapists, the ZeroG was first used as a therapeutic device in 2008. Now in its second iteration, and registered with the Food and Drug Administration (FDA) as a class I medical device, it is available commercially, and the various versions of the device are used in approximately 70 rehabilitation clinics nationwide and at some international sites. The system is mounted to an overhead track, and patients are secured to the machine with a harness with straps that fasten around their shoulders, chest, torso, and bottom. The harness is connected to an overhead spreader bar that is moved along an overhead track by a motorized robotic trolley, which can move at up to 6 mph. The ZeroG has two modes for providing body-weight support: a static body-weight support mode, in which patients can perform limited activities but their position is fixed so they cannot move downward; or dynamic body-weight support mode, in which patients can move up and down, for example from kneeling to standing. The device can support up to 181 kg (~400 lb) in the static mode and provide 4.5kg to 91 kg (~10 to 200 lb) of support in the dynamic mode. Therapists can select different training sessions on a touchscreen or using a wireless remote. The ZeroG's

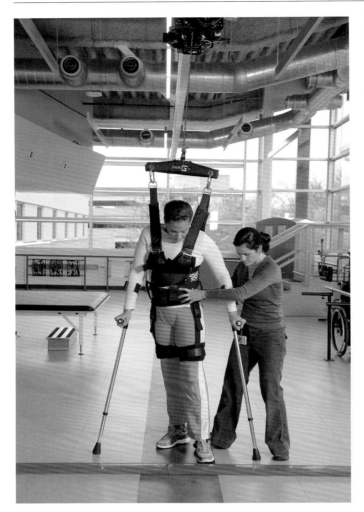

Fig. 13.2 The Aretech ZeroG® used during a therapy session to practice balance. The ZeroG is designed to allow patients with a variety of neurologic impairments to practice walking, balancing, and performing other functional activities while supported by an overhead harness, suspended from a ceiling-mounted track. (Courtesy of Aretech; http://www.aretechllc.com/news-media/photos.)

software system includes interactive target matching and balance games. Games can be set to varying levels of difficulty, together with feedback on balance and postural control in real time. Data from each training session is stored and can be exported in several formats to enable tracking of the patient's progress.

The ZeroG has been studied in persons with stroke, SCI, and cerebral palsy. In a study with 13 able-bodied subjects, Fenuta and Hicks[9] found that electromyogram (EMG) amplitude decreased as body-weight support increased, whereas muscle activation patterns were not significantly altered. Thus, providing body-weight support decreased the intensity of muscular effort required during gait, while allowing generation of normal muscle activation patterns.

Data from SCI studies using ZeroG are currently limited. In a study with patients with incomplete SCI, Fenuta and Hicks[10] determined that the ZeroG did not produce significantly higher lower limb muscle activity in leg muscles studied (tibialis anterior, rectus femoris, biceps femoris, and medial gastrocnemius) compared with using conventional treadmill training. However, the authors suggested that the ZeroG might be useful for more intensive therapy sessions that focus on balance and torso stability, in addition to walking.

The Gait Trainer GT I

The Gait Trainer GT I (Reha-Stim, Berlin, Germany) is an electromechanical device that enables patients to perform task-specific repetitive exercise with less intervention from therapists. It was developed by Drs. Stefan Hesse and Dietmar Uhlenbrock of Klinik Berlin at the Free University of Berlin in Germany,[11] and is designed to simulate a walking gait with a stance/swing phase ratio of 60:40. To accurately simulate gait phases, support for the user's body weight is needed, and the device controls the user's center of mass in horizontal and vertical directions.

Users are secured into the device with a harness; their legs are positioned on two footplates that move backward to simulate the stance phase, and forward to simulate swing phase. The device also consists of two rockers and cranks to propel footplates that the user stands on. Hesse and Uhlenbrock[11] discuss the design specifications. Using the machine, a person's step length and cadence can be continuously adjusted; horizontal and vertical movements that typically occur during the gait cycle are independently controlled by the machine, and a display shows elapsed time, number of steps, velocity, and amount of body-weight support. An optional functional electrical stimulation (FES) system provides four to eight channels to enable stimulation of up to eight nerves or muscles.

Most studies with Gait Trainer GT I till date were either in stroke (subacute or chronic)[12] or in children with Cerebral Palsy.[13] Improved gait function and increased lower-limb muscle activity compared to traditional physical therapy was reported in chronic non-ambulatory stroke subjects.[12] In four independent case studies of persons with incomplete SCI (ASIA C & D), training in GT I with FES improved gait symmetry and dynamic gait pattern. In addition, increases in gait velocity, distance covered, loading of affected limbs and reduction in therapist's effort were reported. It is acknowledged that further controlled clinical studies are warranted.[14] One concern is that the system utilizes continuous foot contact with the supporting footplates, and does not provide inter-mittent sensory input to the plantar skin, as would happen in stance and swing phases of normal gait.

The LOwer extremity Powered Exo Skeleton

The LOwer extremity Powered Exo Skeleton (LOPES) is an impedance-controlled gait training and motor assessment tool developed by researchers at the Department of Biomechanical Engineering of the University of Twente in the Netherlands. The first prototype, developed in 2006, combined a two-dimensional actuated pelvis segment with a leg exoskeleton that had three actuated rotational joints.[15] The device thus combines an exoskeleton—which moves in tandem with the user's legs—with robotic pelvic support, which compensates for the weight of the exoskeleton and enables application of corrective torques to the pelvis. By enabling mechanical interaction between the robot and the patient, this device is designed to provide assistance only as needed; that is, not to hinder movement and provide a continuum of support between two extremes—a "person-in-charge" and "robot-in-charge" modes—in which the device either enables free movement or assists the patient, respectively. Therapists can set the degree of assistance to leg joints and pelvis as required for each user. The LOPES provides eight degrees of freedom (two horizontal degrees for the pelvis and three rotational degrees for each leg), which enables forward walking but also requires some balance control.

Preliminary studies indicated that walking in the device with no robot assistance resembles normal walking.[15] An error–based learning algorithm automatically adjusts the amount of support provided based on the patient's performance in various subtasks, such as foot clearance, which reduces the need for therapist to adjust support.[16] Complementary Limb Motion Estimation (CLME), in which the required movement trajectory for the affected leg is generated based on the normal walking movements of the sound leg, has been incorporated into the machine, and this option increases gait stability and ensures that the amount of support is automatically adapted to the patient's needs.

The device has been studied in stroke survivors since 2008, and there are some data on its use with SCI patients. In an exploratory clinical trial, Fleerkotte et al[17] trained 10 patients with chronic incomplete SCI using the LOPES three times a week for 8 weeks. All participants showed significant improvement in walking speed and distance and in the Walking Index for Spinal Cord Injury, the Six-Minute Walking Test, the Timed Up-and-Go Test, and Lower Extremity Motor Scores. In addition, there was significant improvement in spatiotemporal gait measures and range of motion of the hip. These improvements were maintained at an 8-week follow-up. The authors concluded that the LOPES may improve users' walking ability and quality, in addition to muscle strength. Slow walkers showed the most relative benefit in terms of walking distance and speed.[17]

The PAM/POGO

The PAM/POGO (Biorobotics Laboratory, University of California–Irvine) is a pneumatic robotic device designed to help patients with SCI practice walking on a treadmill, while their body weight is supported, as necessary, by an overhead suspension system. This device comprises a pneumatically operated gait orthosis (POGO) attached to a pelvic assist manipulator (PAM), which assists movement of the pelvis with six actuated degrees of freedom (DOF), allowing unrestricted movement of the pelvis during gait. (Pelvic tilt is unactuated, as this is largely mediated by the body-weight support system, and therapists do not normally provide assistance with this DOF.) POGO, which is worn by the user, provides assistance during the swing phase of gait and prevents knee buckling during stance phase, using a combination of actuated and passive DOF. PAM/POGO enables a full range of natural motion of the legs and pelvis during treadmill walking while providing compliant assistance. Both PAM and POGO are actuated pneumatically; their inherent compliance enables the generation of large forces with lightweight components. Because the PAM enables normal pelvic motion, users can

practice shifting their weight and maintaining balance during walking. Use of compliant assistance means that the user's effort directly impacts the resulting gait, as is the case for unimpaired walking, providing realistic walking practice.[18] Although clinical efficacy has not been determined, this device has shown promising results in preliminary studies to both reduce the demands on therapists during body-weight–supported gait training and to provide realistic stepping practice for individuals with SCI.[18]

Limitations

Robotic gait-training devices hold much promise for providing consistent, quantifiable therapy while reducing the need for multiple therapists and reducing the physical burden on those therapists. However, rational training strategies to optimize locomotor recovery in individuals with incomplete SCI using such devices have yet to be established. Further barriers to clinical acceptance of these tools include potential high cost and large size, technical complexity, and safety concerns, all of which limit robot implementation in clinical settings and preclude their use at home. Furthermore, their size and cost mean that rigorous randomized controlled trials are difficult to implement, so that full-scale validation of their therapeutic value remains difficult to achieve, and has not been fully accomplished to date.

■ Wearable Robotic Devices

More recently, wearable robotic or exoskeleton devices have been used to compensate for impaired lower limb function in patients with both complete and incomplete SCI. Unlike treadmill-based therapies, these devices offer the possibility of providing over-ground mobility in addition to therapeutic applications. Many of these devices have been designed for therapeutic purposes, although some are now offering mobility assistance for home and community use. Currently, there are four devices commercially available for therapeutic use and one for personal mobility use. However, 15 to 20 different types of exoskeleton will be ready to enter the market in the next 2 to 5 years. These devices differ in some of their structural framework, but they all provide stability for walking through lower extremity bracing, sensors that detect a user's desired movements and motors or actuators that operate the device. Research for both therapy and mobility applications is limited and warrants longer-term investigation.

The ReWalk

The ReWalk™ (ReWalk Robotics, Inc., Marlboro, MA, and Yokneam Illit, Israel) is a lower-limb exoskeleton with bilateral hip and knee joint actuator motors, powered by rechargeable batteries, to assist individuals with SCI to stand upright, walk, and ascend and descend ramps, curbs, and stairs (**Fig. 13.3**). The stairs function is not FDA approved and so at present, use of stairs can be undertaken only in research settings. For all other functionalities, this device has FDA clearance for personal use for injuries at levels T7-L5 (although a trained caregiver must accompany the user at all times due to the risk of falling). The device is also approved for therapeutic use in the clinic for levels T4-L5. This device is currently the only exoskeleton with FDA clearance for personal use (although a trained caregiver must accompany the user at all times due to the risk of falling). Sensors measure upper-body tilt angle, joint angles, and ground contact.[19] The ReWalk is adjusted to fit the user, and Velcro straps around the trunk, waist, thighs, knees, and calves secure the user into the device; users' feet are placed over the footplates. Forearm crutches ensure stability, provide additional comfort and safety, and help the user sense the ground.[19] Users wear a backpack that contains the control system and batteries, and additional padding can be used to improve comfort and to reduce the risk of skin injury.

A wireless remote controller worn on the wrist is used to select different sitting, standing, or walking modes, and users operate the ReWalk through minimal movements of the trunk to change the center of gravity. To initi-

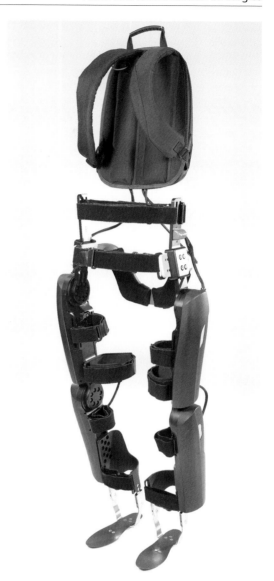

Fig. 13.3 The ReWalk is a lower-limb exoskeleton designed to assist individuals with lower extremity weakness due to spinal cord injury (SCI) to stand upright, walk, and ascend and descend stairs. (Courtesy of ReWalk Robotics, Inc.)

ate the first step in walking mode, users must lean their trunk forward until a tilt sensor located on the lateral trunk support detects an 8-degree change in sagittal plane position. This event initiates a preset hip and knee displacement, resulting in leg swing. The user then returns the trunk to an upright position to complete the swing phase and ensure toe clearance. Joint angle displacements for the knee and hip can be adjusted using an external computer to optimize the walking characteristics or implement a training mode. The tilt sensor can be bypassed in a manual mode, which can be used for sit-to-stand transitions.[19]

The ReWalk is produced in two versions: the ReWalk Rehabilitation is designed for therapeutic purposes, and the ReWalk Personal is designed for mobility in the home and community. Patients with lower extremity paralysis or paresis due to SCI level T7 to L5 can use the device in the home and community setting, when accompanied by a trained caregiver; those with lesions at levels T4 to T6 are restricted to a rehabilitation setting.[20] Users must have adequate bilateral upper limb strength, trunk control, and lower limb length, and must have sufficient range of motion in the lower extremity to allow for ambulation. They must tolerate upright positioning and walking without experiencing adverse autonomic effects, and have adequate bone density.

In one study, after training with the ReWalk, 12 nonambulatory patients with thoracic-level motor-complete SCI were able to walk continuously using the device without additional assistance for at least 50 to 100 m, and for periods of at least 5 to 10 minutes at speeds of 0.03 to 0.45 m/s.[19] The device was safe to use, with no serious adverse effects observed. Additional beneficial effects in other areas included improved bowel and bladder function, reduced spasticity, and improved pain levels.

The Ekso

The Ekso™ (Ekso Bionics, Berkeley, CA) is a lower-extremity exoskeleton intended for use as a gait training tool for patients with lower extremity weakness following SCI (motor complete paralysis C7 or below; incomplete SCI with functional bilateral upper extremity strength or functional strength of one upper extremity and one lower extremity) or other neurologic injury with similar outcome. The FDA has approved the use of the Ekso in the clinical

setting for individuals with SCI and stroke. A unique feature of the Ekso is the variable assist program, which allows therapists to adjust how much assistance the device provides at the hip and knee, based on the user's ability. The Ekso, which weighs 50 lb, comprises two upper and lower leg segments that can be adjusted to fit the user, that is, to align the user's joints with the Ekso joints. These limb segments are connected to a rigid torso structure, which also contains the computer and batteries. Four motors actuate the hip and knee joints in the sagittal plane.[21] The therapist can control the device, and settings are adjusted to meet the user's evolving needs.

The Ekso has three functions—sit-to-stand, walk, and stand-to-sit—and three walking modes: (1) FirstStep, in which the trained therapist controls the device. (2) ProStep, in which users achieve the next step by moving their hips forward and shifting them laterally; the Ekso recognizes that the user is in the correct position and takes the steps. (3) ProStep Plus, in which the device is triggered not only by weight shift but also by forward leg movement. Although the Ekso™ provides external stability, patients must practice static and dynamic standing balance activities to ensure they can maintain their balance, before walking in the device using an appropriate assistive device.

Using the Ekso, some patients with SCI demonstrated improvements in walking speed and balance, though larger clinical trials are needed. In a prospective pilot study, Kolakowsky-Hayner et al[22] evaluated the feasibility and safety of using the Ekso to aid individuals with SCI (complete TI or below) with ambulation, and found the device safe for use in a controlled environment with a trained professional.

The Indego

The Indego® (Parker Hannifin Corp., Macedonia, OH) is a lower extremity exoskeleton designed to enable patients with lower extremity weakness following SCI to stand, walk, and perform stand-to-sit and sit-to-stand transitions (**Fig. 13.4**). The FDA has approved the Indego for personal use by individuals with spinal cord

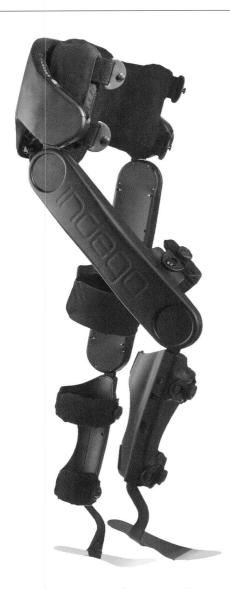

Fig. 13.4 The Indego is a lower extremity exoskeleton designed to enable individuals with lower extremity weakness or paralysis due to SCI and other conditions to stand, walk, and perform stand-to-sit transitions. (Courtesy of Parker Hannifin.)

and lower leg segments and a hip segment—that are available in three sizes. Due to this modular design, the device can be assembled while a patient is seated. A rechargeable lithium-ion battery and electronics are housed in the hip segment, and the upper leg segments contain the actuation units and electronics. The lower leg segments contain ankle foot orthoses that attach to the upper leg segments at the knee. A wireless controller enables the therapist to control the device, and to capture and export data.

The Indego has three operational modes—sit, stand, and walk—in addition to standby (pause) modes and a "Go!" mode, which enables the user to transition between modes. All movements are controlled by shifts in the user's body weight and changes in body position. The device is intended for users with complete or incomplete SCI level C5 or lower. Users must have adequate passive range of motion at their shoulders, hips, knees, and ankles, and sufficient upper body strength to safely use a crutch support system. In a pilot study involving 16 patients with SCI and injury levels ranging from L1 incomplete to C5 complete, all participants were able to walk indoors and out of doors after five 1.5-hour training sessions with the Indego.[23] Walking speeds and distances achieved suggested that the Indego could enable some individuals with SCI to become limited community ambulators.

The REX

The REX (Rex Bionics Ltd., Auckland, New Zealand) is designed for patients with mobility impairments, including complete SCI up to the C4-C5 level. The REX Personal (REX P) is designed for home use.[24] Unlike other exoskeletons, the REX is self-balancing and a walking frame or crutches are not required,[24] possibly reducing adverse impact on shoulders. The device is controlled by the user with a joystick. Although the REX has five actuated degrees of freedom that enable the user to sit, stand, and turn, it is a relatively large, heavy exoskeleton, and may not enable adequate voluntary limb exercise in its current form.

injuries at levels T7-L5, and rehabilitation use for patients at injury levels T4-L5. The device, which weighs 12kg (~26 lb), is designed to be used with forearm crutches or other devices that assist with stability. The Indego comprises five modular components—right and left upper

The HAL

The HAL® (Hybrid Assistive Limb; Cyberdyne Inc., Tsukuba, Japan) is a full-body exoskeleton originally developed to assist the elderly and to help individuals with disabilities walk, climb stairs, and lift objects. The HAL comprises power units and angle sensors for the upper and lower limbs, a floor reaction force sensor, a control unit on the back, and bioelectric signal sensors embedded in the device that detect EMG signals on the user's skin surface to predict the user's intended movements.[25] The HAL combines an EMG-based control system with a robotic autonomous controller that generates gait patterns to control the device, which can assist with walking and sit-to-stand transitions.[26]

The Exo-H2

The Exo-H2 (Technaid S.L., Madrid, Spain) is a lower limb robotic exoskeleton with an open control architecture that enables the user to modify and adjust control parameters to optimize the system for the user. It has been used primarily in a research setting to date.

Limitations

These new exoskeletons are an important innovation, and raise hopes that many patients with mobility impairments due to SCI and other conditions can return to standing and walking in the home and community, and achieve a greater level of independence. However, there is limited evidence to date that they are a safe and effective form of locomotor training for rehabilitation therapy. (A trained therapist or caregiver must monitor the user constantly.) This is likely because the gait achieved is quite halting and intermittent, and relies heavily on safe placement of the assistive device, limiting continuity of motion, and total locomotor step dosage. It is unlikely, therefore, that exoskeletons will provide a competitive alternative to treadmill training using a robotic gait trainer or even manual gait training for therapeutic purposes, at least in the near term. However, more intuitive controllers in the exoskeletons that enable continuous stepping and other activities such as climbing stairs or ramps, or training on dynamic stability and balance, may increase the potential of these devices as therapeutic tools. Furthermore, other training strategies such as functional electrical stimulation or spinal stimulation, which when combined with exoskeleton training seem to enhance functional benefits, are still being evaluated.

■ Upper Limb Robotic Trainers

Many of these devices were developed for rehabilitation of arm movement after stroke, which is the primary cause of upper limb movement disorders. Furthermore, most clinical studies have been done in stroke survivors or in healthy subjects, with a few studies in other populations with impaired upper limb function, such as multiple sclerosis, Guillain-Barré syndrome, and SCI.

The InMotion ARM Robot

The InMotion ARM™ Robot (Interactive Motion Technologies, Watertown, MA) is the clinical version of the MIT-Manus, an impedance-controlled robotic arm with two degrees of freedom, which uses intelligent, interactive technology to provide intensive therapy that continuously adapts to and challenges each patient. The patient sits at a table, putting his/her lower arm and wrist into a brace attached to the arm of the robot. A video screen prompts the patient to perform an arm exercise, and if the patient is unable to move the arm, the device moves it. If the patient is able to move the arm, the robot provides adjustable levels of guidance and assistance to facilitate this movement, providing little or no resistance to enable weak users to move the device. This end-effector design is easy to don and doff, and is effective for joint angle changes of 45 degrees of less.

In a clinical trial of stroke survivors who received an hour of training with the MIT-Manus in addition to conventional therapy, measures of increased movement were twice as high as for patients who received "sham" robotic therapy (i.e., the robot was attached to the patient but did not assist with movement). These improvements were sustained at 3-year follow up.[27] Although studies in SCI are limited, a pilot study was conducted in nine patients with incomplete spinal injuries, levels C4 to C6, sustained 2 years or longer before the study. Patients received treatment on the InMotion ARM robot for 18 sessions over 6 weeks, with one arm followed by the same training with the other arm. A sample of two patients exhibited greater than 10% changes in Fugl-Meyer scores and 20% changes in the Motor Power Scales, and although both arms were trained separately, similar gains were obtained in both.

The Armeo Spring

The Armeo® Spring (Hocoma Inc., Norwell, MA, and Volketswil, Switzerland) was derived from an elegant passive arm support system developed for use in children with muscular dystrophy at DuPont Hospital in Delaware (**Fig. 13.5**). It was redesigned for adult use as a Therapy Wilmington Robotic Exoskeleton (T-WREX) by David Reinkensmeyer, PhD, at the University of California, Irvine (UCI) and the Rehabilitation Institute of Chicago (RIC). The Armeo Spring, as it is now called, is a passive (i.e., non-actuated) arm orthosis that provides adjustable arm support and is sensorized to measure

arm movement and hand grasp as users interact with computer games.

Passive devices, such as the Armeo Spring, are likely to be less costly and to pose fewer safety concerns than robotic actuated devices and so can be used semi-independently. Furthermore, the device does not provide any assistance with movement; thus arm movement requires increased effort and attention from the user, potentially contributing to an enhanced therapeutic benefit.

The arm support enables users with a moderate to severe impairment to achieve a large active range of motion of arm movement, and enables them to begin to use their hand in meaningful ways. Even small arm movements can be detected by electronic movement and handgrip force sensors, and can be used to control computer games and provide quantitative feedback to the user and clinician. The Armeo enables users to work in a three-dimensional workspace and is adjustable for different limb sizes. An extensive library of game-like software enables users to perform exercises in a virtual-reality environment, which displays the functional task and provides instant performance feedback. Exercises target both distal and proximal arm movements, including grasp and release, pronation and supination of the arm, extension and flexion of the wrist, and reaching and retrieving functions. The exercises are designed to assess motor ability and coordination, and sensors record arm and joint

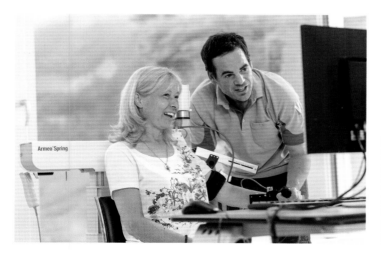

Fig. 13.5 The Armeo® Spring is a passive arm orthosis that provides adjustable arm support. It measures arm movement and hand grasps as users interact with computer games. (Courtesy of Hocoma, Volketswil, Switzerland.)

movements, which can be accessed to document progress and set clinical goals.

Although this device has not been formally evaluated in SCI, a pilot study with the T-WREX indicated that 8 weeks of training significantly improved arm movement ability for individuals with moderate to severe hemiparesis following severe stroke.[28] Other studies in stroke patients further demonstrated that the T-WREX provided a small but significant reduction in impairment compared with conventional therapy at 6-month follow-up. Although, this finding may not have had functional significance these gains were similar to those achieved using actuated robotic devices. However, users preferred the T-WREX over conventional therapy, which may increase compliance. Additionally, an 8-week training program in which the Armeo Spring was used to supplement conventional therapy in 10 individuals with severe multiple sclerosis showed significant improvement in functional tests at the end of treatment, and function improved further at 2-month follow-up, suggesting that participants used their arm more following treatment.[29]

Limitations

Upper extremity exoskeletons offer promise as therapeutic devices by enabling more extensive practice and engaging trainee interest. They can be programmed to highlight certain aspects of rehabilitation training, and appear to be a useful addition to the therapeutic toolbox of the physical or occupational therapy team. Although offering promise as devices to augment neural plasticity, their use is limited by the lack of a coherent therapeutic framework, and treatments are thus somewhat ad hoc in flavor.

■ Wearable Sensors

Assessing the efficacy of advanced rehabilitation technology for patients with SCI requires robust outcome measures that accurately evaluate changes in ability. Traditional outcome measures may assess physical ability, such as number of steps taken or gait speed at a single point, like a snapshot. However, quantification of advanced robotic technologies requires continuous monitoring of stepping practice or gait speed at a high resolution and evaluating other important aspects of rehabilitation and recovery, including physiological and psychological changes, which are essential to well-being and an enhanced quality of life.[30] A variety of novel sensors are now available to monitor stepping or activities within the community. Commercially available devices include wrist sensors such as Fitbit, Jawbone, Nike+ FuelBand, and smart watches from companies like Samsung, TAG HEUER, and Apple. The monitoring capabilities of these commercial sensors are limited currently by their ability to sensitively monitor only healthy people, whereas performance is under- or overestimated in SCI patients. Research-based sensors, however, have been tested extensively in the SCI population. Two such sensors have been tested in the SCI population:

The StepWatch Activity Monitor

The StepWatch Activity Monitor (SAM) (Modus Health LLC, Washington DC), is a wearable step counter that uses acceleration-based algorithms to evaluate steps and provide an accurate profile of daily activity. It has been shown to be accurate at slow walking speeds, and when worn on the ankle of either the affected or less affected limb. Studies in patients with SCI demonstrated that 2 days of monitoring using the StepWatch was sufficient to obtain reliable data on daily stepping activity and locomotor activity.[31]

The ActiGraph wGT3X-BT Device

The ActiGraph wGT3X-BT device (ActiGraph LLC, Pensacola, FL) uses accelerometer technology to monitor activity—from sleep to ambulation—and software that uses validated algorithms to interpret that activity (**Fig. 13.6**). It also uses a gyroscope to measure nonambulatory movement or to detect falls; a proximity meter to

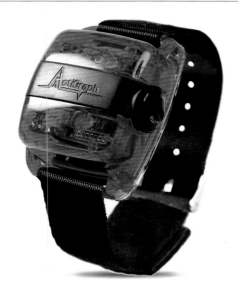

Fig. 13.6 The ActiGraph wGT3X-BT device uses accelerometer technology to monitor activity, and has software that uses validated algorithms to interpret that activity. It has been used to monitor physical activity and energy expenditure in wheelchair users with SCI. (Courtesy of ActiGraph.)

measure social interactions; and an inclinometer to determine whether the subject is sitting, standing, or lying down. The ActiGraph wGT3X-BT can also provide heart-rate monitoring when augmented with an additional heart-rate monitor. It can provide estimates of average metabolic rates, energy expenditure, intensity of physical activity, and amount of sedentary behavior. It can also evaluate sleep quality and quantity. The ActiGraph provides real-time access to data through Bluetooth® technology and cloud data storage. The Acti-Graph has been used to monitor physical activity[32] and energy expenditure[33] in wheelchair users with SCI.

Limitations

The introduction of lightweight sensors in the field of neurologic rehabilitation is an exciting addition to efforts attempting to establish quantitative, continuous, and sensitive monitoring of clinical outcome parameters in patients with disabling neurologic disorders,

such as SCI. This enables researchers to monitor, intervene, and then continue to monitor the use of advanced technologies both for therapeutic and mobility purposes. When patients are not meeting their target results, clinicians can thus address these issues in an almost real-time response, resulting in a better ability to modify the hardware or controller of these advanced technologies to suit the needs of the individual patient. The major barriers experienced currently are that these devices generate large volumes of data for the clinician to review, synthesize, and understand, which is burdensome. It is currently impractical for most clinicians to use precious therapy time to review the extensive outcomes data provided by these sensors. What is needed, then, is a way to synthesize sensor data into a convenient and compact numerical form that can be seen as equivalent to prevailing clinical measures.

▪ Conclusion

Advanced technologies targeting both therapeutic and mobility objectives are rapidly emerging in the field of neurologic rehabilitation. Some emerging rehabilitation technologies designed for individuals with SCI include treadmill-based robotic trainers; wearable robotic devices, including exoskeletons; upper-limb robotic trainers; and lightweight sensors that assist in establishing quantitative clinical outcome parameters. These devices may reduce the physical demands on therapists during training sessions, and may be used alongside other advanced training strategies to enhance their functional benefits. Although these technologies hold much promise, validated rehabilitation protocols for these devices have yet to be developed. For some current devices, high cost, large size, and safety concerns may preclude their use outside of the clinic. Significant research is needed to evaluate the long-term potential of these devices in larger studies, to devise standardized therapeutic protocols for specific target populations, and to reduce the size and cost of these devices.

Chapter Summary

Traumatic SCI is a devastating medical condition that can adversely influence a person's quality of life and ability to live independently. However, as emergency care and rehabilitation protocols for persons with SCI have improved in recent decades, several advanced engineering and robotic technologies to assist and augment therapist actions have also emerged. These technologies are aimed at improving upper-limb strength and function. Treadmill-based robotic devices and exoskeletons allow individuals to practice balancing and walking, as well as to perform other functional activities. Although these devices may reduce the need for multiple therapists during therapy sessions, training strategies to optimize locomotor recovery in robotic trainers and exoskeletons have yet to be realized, and their high cost may prevent use outside of the clinic. The wearer's safety when using an untethered exoskeleton also remains a significant concern. Similarly, upper extremity exoskeletal devices may allow patients more extensive practice in training exercises, but their use is limited by the lack of a coherent framework for therapy. Finally, wearable sensors are also being developed to help researchers establish quantitative clinical outcome parameters in persons with neurologic conditions such as SCI. All of these devices offer great potential to improve the quality of life and enhance recovery in persons with SCI. However, due to several limitations, it may take several more years of research before the full capability of these technologies is realized.

Pearls

- Several emerging technologies, such as robotic trainers and exoskeletons, have the potential to enhance the recovery and quality of life for individuals with traumatic SCI.
- Robotic gait-training devices may provide consistent, quantifiable therapy for persons with incomplete SCI while reducing the need for multiple therapists during therapy sessions.
- Lower limb exoskeletons have the potential to help individuals with SCI or other conditions maintain neuromuscular health through over-ground locomotor training, and enable them to stand and walk in their home or community.
- Upper extremity exoskeletons may provide patients extensive practice in training exercises.
- Wearable sensors may aid researchers in establishing quantitative clinical outcome parameters to more accurately evaluate changes in ability in persons with SCI or other neuromuscular impairments.

Pitfalls

- Specific training protocols to optimize locomotor recovery in robotic trainers and exoskeletons have not yet been established.
- To date, there is limited evidence indicating that exoskeletons are safe and effective for community mobility.
- Data on the effectiveness of upper limb trainers are not well developed.
- Many lower extremity devices are large and heavy, as well as costly, which may preclude their use outside of the clinic.
- Current wearable sensors produce large volumes of data, and it may be impractical for clinicians to spend their time mining through such large amounts of information.

References

Five Must-Read References

1. Anderson KD. Targeting recovery: priorities of the spinal cord-injured population. J Neurotrauma 2004;21:1371–1383
2. Courtine G, Gerasimenko Y, van den Brand R, et al. Transformation of nonfunctional spinal circuits into functional states after the loss of brain input. Nat Neurosci 2009;12:1333–1342
3. Behrman AL, Lawless-Dixon AR, Davis SB, et al. Locomotor training progression and outcomes after incomplete spinal cord injury. Phys Ther 2005;85:1356–1371
4. History of Hocoma. 2015. http://www.hocoma.com/en/about-us/company/history/. Accessed July 29, 2015
5. Wirz M, Zemon DH, Rupp R, et al. Effectiveness of automated locomotor training in patients with chronic incomplete spinal cord injury: a multicenter trial. Arch Phys Med Rehabil 2005;86:672–680

6. Hornby TG, Zemon DH, Campbell D. Robotic-assisted, body-weight-supported treadmill training in individuals following motor incomplete spinal cord injury. Phys Ther 2005;85:52–66

7. Shin JC, Kim JY, Park HK, Kim NY. Effect of robotic-assisted gait training in patients with incomplete spinal cord injury. Ann Rehabil Med 2014;38:719–725

8. Hidler J, Brennan D, Black I, Nichols D, Brady K, Nef T. ZeroG: overground gait and balance training system. J Rehabil Res Dev 2011;48:287–298

9. Fenuta AM, Hicks AL. Muscle activation during body weight-supported locomotion while using the ZeroG. J Rehabil Res Dev 2014;51:51–58

10. Fenuta AM, Hicks AL. Metabolic demand and muscle activation during different forms of bodyweight supported locomotion in men with incomplete SCI. Biomed Res Int 2014;2014:632765

11. Hesse S, Uhlenbrock D. A mechanized gait trainer for restoration of gait. J Rehabil Res Dev 2000;37:701–708

12. Pohl M, Werner C, Holzgraefe M, et al. Repetitive locomotor training and physiotherapy improve walking and basic activities of daily living after stroke: a single-blind, randomized multicentre trial (DEutsche GAngtrainerStudie, DEGAS). Clin Rehabil 2007;21:17–27

13. Smania N, Bonetti P, Gandolfi M, et al. Improved gait after repetitive locomotor training in children with cerebral palsy. Am J Phys Med Rehabil 2011;90:137–149

14. Hesse S, Werner C, Bardeleben A. Electromechanical gait training with functional electrical stimulation: case studies in spinal cord injury. Spinal Cord 2004;42:346–352

15. Veneman JF, Kruidhof R, Hekman EE, Ekkelenkamp R, Van Asseldonk EH, van der Kooij H. Design and evaluation of the LOPES exoskeleton robot for interactive gait rehabilitation. IEEE Trans Neural Syst Rehabil Eng 2007;15:379–386

16. van Asseldonk E, Koopman B, Buurke JH, Simons C, van der Kooij H. Selective and adaptive robotic support of foot clearance for training stroke survivors with stiff knee gait. 2009 IEEE 11th International Conference on Rehabilitation Robotics. Kyoto International Conference Center, Japan, June 23–26, 2009: 602–607

17. Fleerkotte BM, Koopman B, Buurke JH, van Asseldonk EH, van der Kooij H, Rietman JS. The effect of impedance-controlled robotic gait training on walking ability and quality in individuals with chronic incomplete spinal cord injury: an explorative study. J Neuroeng Rehabil 2014;11:26

18. Aoyagi D, Ichinose WE, Harkema SJ, Reinkensmeyer DJ, Bobrow JE. A robot and control algorithm that can synchronously assist in naturalistic motion during body-weight-supported gait training following neurologic injury. IEEE Trans Neural Syst Rehabil Eng 2007;15:387–400

19. Esquenazi A, Talaty M, Packel A, Saulino M. The ReWalk powered exoskeleton to restore ambulatory function to individuals with thoracic-level motor-complete spinal cord injury. Am J Phys Med Rehabil 2012;91:911–921

20. FDA Allows Marketing of First Wearable Motorized Device that Helps People with Certain Spinal Cord Injuries to Walk [press release]. fda.gov, 2014. http://www.fda.gov/NewsEvents/Newsroom/PressAnnouncements/ucm402970.htm

21. Kressler J, Thomas CK, Field-Fote EC, et al. Understanding therapeutic benefits of overground bionic ambulation: exploratory case series in persons with chronic, complete spinal cord injury. Arch Phys Med Rehabil 2014;95:1878–1887.e4

22. Kolakowsky-Hayner S, Crew J, Moran S, Shah A. Safety and feasibility of using the Ekso Bionic Exoskeleton to aid ambulation after spinal cord injury. J Spine. 2013 doi.org/10.4172/2165-7939.S4-003

23. Hartigan C, Kandilakis C, Dalley S, et al. Mobility outcomes following five training sessions with a powered exoskeleton. Top Spinal Cord Inj Rehabil 2015; 21:93–99

24. REX Bionics—Our Products. 2015. http://www.rexbionics.com/products/. Accessed May 28, 2015

25. Bogue R. Exoskeletons and robotic prosthetics: a review of recent developments. Industrial robot. Ind Robot 2009;36:421–427

26. Kawamoto H, Taal S, Niniss H, et al. Voluntary motion support control of Robot Suit HAL triggered by bio-electrical signal for hemiplegia. Conference proceedings: Annual International Conference of the IEEE Engineering in Medicine and Biology Society. 2010: 462–466

27. Volpe BT, Krebs HI, Hogan N, Edelsteinn L, Diels CM, Aisen ML. Robot training enhanced motor outcome in patients with stroke maintained over 3 years. Neurology 1999;53:1874–1876

28. Sanchez RJ, Liu J, Rao S, et al. Automating arm movement training following severe stroke: functional exercises with quantitative feedback in a gravity-reduced environment. IEEE Trans Neural Syst Rehabil Eng 2006;14:378–389

29. Gijbels D, Lamers I, Kerkhofs L, Alders G, Knippenberg E, Feys P. The Armeo Spring as training tool to improve upper limb functionality in multiple sclerosis: a pilot study. J Neuroeng Rehabil 2011; 8:5

30. Bowden MG, Hannold EM, Nair PM, Fuller LB, Behrman AL. Beyond gait speed: a case report of a multidimensional approach to locomotor rehabilitation outcomes in incomplete spinal cord injury. J Neurol Phys Ther 2008;32:129–138

31. Ishikawa S, Stevens SL, Kang M, Morgan DW. Reliability of daily step activity monitoring in adults with incomplete spinal cord injury. J Rehabil Res Dev 2011;48:1187–1194

32. Warms CA, Belza BL. Actigraphy as a measure of physical activity for wheelchair users with spinal cord injury. Nurs Res 2004;53:136–143

33. García-Massó X, Serra-Añó P, García-Raffi LM, Sánchez-Pérez EA, López-Pascual J, Gonzalez LM. Validation of the use of Actigraph GT3X accelerometers to estimate energy expenditure in full time manual wheelchair users with spinal cord injury. Spinal Cord 2013;51:898–903

Brain–Computer Interfaces to Enhance Function After Spinal Cord Injury

Rüdiger Rupp

Introduction

It is estimated that 300,000 people in Europe and the United States are currently living with the consequences of spinal cord injury (SCI), with 11,000 new injuries occurring each year. Currently, 55% of individuals with SCI are tetraplegic due to injuries of the cervical spinal cord; 28% of all patients with SCI have a neurologic level of lesion of C4 or C5 at the time of discharge from acute care to rehabilitation facilities.[1] In this patient group at least some residual capabilities for manipulation of objects are still preserved. About 8% of all patients have a neurologic level rostral to C4, resulting in the severe impairment of motor functions of both upper extremities, including the shoulder and elbow, as well as hand movements. Surveys among people with tetraplegia have reported that although a high level of user satisfaction has already been achieved, there is a need for better assistive technology solutions to help with manipulation, mobility, communication, electronic entertainment, and environmental control.[2,3] Modern life cannot be imagined without computer access. Access to the Internet and social media platforms is even more important for people with severe motor impairments, because the virtual world enables people with handicaps to function on a par with the able-bodied. Depending on the residual capabilities of the impaired user, joysticks for the hand or the chin, suck-and-puff control, voice control, or eye-tracking systems can serve as user interfaces for control of assistive technology. In patients with a very high spinal lesion, only a few electronic user interfaces are available, and even those that are applicable may not enable a sufficient level of performance over an extended period of time. Therefore, over the last decade, brain–computer interfaces (BCIs) have become an interesting option for impaired users who achieve only a moderate level of control with traditional input devices or quickly become physically fatigued.

Noninvasive Brain–Computer Interfaces

The BCIs are technical systems that provide a direct connection between the human brain and assistive technology.[4] These systems are able to detect thought-modulated changes in electrophysiological brain activity and transform the changes into control signals. A BCI system consists of five sequential components: (1) signal acquisition; (2) feature extraction; (3) feature translation; (4) classification output, which interfaces to an output device; and (5) feedback to the user, provided by the output device. Although all implementations of BCIs build on the same basic components, they differ substantially in regard to the degree of invasiveness, the complexity of the hardware

Table 14.1 An Overview of the Most Common Practical Types of Electroencephalogram (EEG)-Based Brain–Computer Interfaces (BCIs)

BCI	Minimal (typical) Number of Electrodes	Qualitative Estimation of Typical Training Time	Population with 90–100% (Below 80%) Accuracy Without Training	Typical Rate of Decisions per Minute
SMR (2-class)	4 (10) + 1 reference + 1 ground	Weeks to months	6% (81%)	4 bits/min
P300	3 (9) + 1 reference + 1 ground	Minutes to < 1 hour	73% (11%)	10 bits/min
SSVEP	6 +1 reference + 1 ground	Minutes to < 1 hour	87% (4%)	12 bits/min

Abbreviations: SMR, sensorimotor rhythm; SSVEP, steady-state visual evoked potential.

and software components, the basic mode of operation (cue-based, synchronous versus asynchronous), and the underlying physiological mechanisms.[5] Noninvasive BCIs represent the first choice in user applications due to their ease of application. Although a variety of different data acquisition methods can be used for the setup of a BCI, such as functional magnetic resonance imaging (fMRI), near-infrared spectroscopy (NIRS), and magnetoencephalography (MEG), most noninvasive systems rely on brain signals that are recorded by electrodes on the scalp (electroencephalogram, EEG). EEG-based BCI systems can function in most environments with relatively small and inexpensive equipment, and therefore offer the potential for everyday use at home.

A variety of EEG signals have been used as measures of brain activity: event-related potentials (ERPs), steady-state visual evoked potentials (SSVEP), and frequency oscillations such as sensorimotor rhythms (SMRs). EEG-based BCI systems can be categorized as endogenous (synonym: asynchronous) or exogenous (synonym: synchronous). Asynchronous BCIs depend on the users' ability to voluntary modulate their electrophysiological activity such as the EEG amplitude in a specific frequency band. In asynchronous BCIs, the time point for changes of the control signals is not predefined by the system, but the user is free to initiate decisions at any time. These systems usually require a substantial amount of training. Examples of this class of BCIs are systems based on the detection of SMRs. Synchronous BCIs depend on the electrophysiological activity evoked by external

stimuli and do not require intensive training. The most common synchronous BCI is based on P300 event-related potentials. Although systems based on steady-state evoked potentials such as SSVEPs combine components of asynchronous and synchronous approaches, the introduction of cues improves their accuracy. Depending on the brain signals used for operation, BCIs greatly vary in regard to the minimal and typically used number of electrodes, training times, accuracies, and typical information transfer rates (**Table 14.1**). At the current state of the art, all noninvasive BCIs have a significantly lower performance level than manual input devices like joysticks, computer mouses, or keyboards. Therefore, a BCI represents only an alternative in end users, who are generally not able to operate such devices or cannot use these devices over a prolonged period of time.

■ BCIs Based on Event-Related Potentials

Event-related potential (ERP)-based BCIs make use of the fact that specific neural activity is triggered by and involved in the processing of specific events. These systems are implemented with an oddball paradigm, wherein a rare target (oddball event) is presented within frequent nontarget events. These BCIs usually exploit an endogenous ERP component, known as P300, as input signal. The P300 is a positive deflection in the EEG occurring 200 to 500 milliseconds after the presentation of the rare visual, auditory, or somatosensory stimulus, and is a reliable, easy-to-detect, event-related potential. By focusing attention on the rare target, such as by keeping a mental count of its occurrence, the P300 amplitude can be increased, and therefore its detection and classification improves.[6] In individuals with SCI, eye-gaze is preserved, and thus a visual rather than an auditory oddball paradigm is the preferred choice. The information transfer rate and accuracy are substantially higher and the perceived workload is much lower in visual P300-based BCIs than in other ERP-based BCIs. The big advantage of P300-based BCIs compared with SMR-based BCIs is that they can be operated with almost no training in 99% of the general population.

BCIs Based on Steady-State Evoked Potentials

Steady-state evoked potentials (SSEPs) are stable oscillations that can be elicited by rapid repetitive (usually > 6 repetitions per second) visual, auditory, or sensory stimuli. The most common type of SSEP-based BCIs is the SSVEP-based BCI, in which screen objects flickering at different frequencies are visually presented to subjects. Focusing their attention on the intended stimulus elicits enhanced SSVEP responses at the corresponding frequency, which can be detected, classified, and translated into control commands. SSVEP-based BCIs have several advantages: they employ a high information transfer rate, they require only minimal training, and they work in almost every user. SSVEP-BCIs are the preferred choice in individuals with SCI and unimpaired visual function, because the information transfer rate of BCIs based on auditory steady-state responses is 10-fold lower than that of SSVEP-based systems.

BCIs Based on Sensorimotor Rhythms

One type of EEG-based BCIs exploits the modulation of SMRs. These rhythms are oscillations in the EEG occurring in the α/mu (8–12 Hz) and/or β (18–26 Hz) bands and can be recorded over the primary sensorimotor areas on the scalp. Although the mu-rhythm is more pronounced in the EEG during "idling" (event-related synchronization [ERD]), its amplitude typically decreases (event-related desynchronization) during actual movement and similarly during mental rehearsal of movements (motor imagery [MI]). It has been shown that able-bodied people can learn to modulate the SMR amplitude by practicing MIs of simple movements (e.g., hand/foot movements).[7] This process occurs in a closed loop, meaning that the system recognizes the SMR amplitude changes evoked by MI, and these changes are instantaneously fed back to the users. This neurofeedback procedure together with mutual human-machine adaptation normally enables BCI users after some weeks of training to control their SMR activity and use these modulations to control output devices in an asynchronous, self-paced manner. With SMR-BCIs, a sophisticated level of control (e.g., a three-dimensional cursor control) can be achieved.[8]

Although BCIs based on the registration of P300 and SSVEPs can be operated by a vast majority of users, SMR-BCIs cannot. In the SMR-based BCI approach, in up to one third of the non–motor-impaired participants the BCI is unable to detect classifiable, task-related EEG patterns. Consequently, these subjects cannot quickly be provided with a BCI-controlled application or need at least a substantial amount of training to reach a sufficient level of performance. The causes of this inability to control a BCI (another synonym of this low BCI aptitude is "BCI-inefficiency") have not yet been satisfactorily determined. Most of the experiments on the gain in performance with training in SMR-BCIs were performed in able-bodied subjects, and so it is unclear to what extent these results can be applied to persons with SCI. In a single case study, in which an individual with a lesion of the upper cervical spinal cord was provided with a BCI-controlled upper extremity neuroprosthesis, no positive training effects occurred in a training period of more than 6 months. Even after 415 MI-BCI runs, the user's average performance did not show any trend toward improvement, but remained at ~ 70%

with large day-to-day variances.[9] This confounding factor, among others, represents a challenge for successful use of SMR-BCIs.[10]

For a typical two-class SMR-BCI, different paradigms of MIs, such as one hand versus the feet or left versus right hand, are used either in a switch-based ("brain switch") fashion by introduction of a threshold or in an analog manner by directly connecting the classifier output to the output device. An often underestimated problem in practical applications of BCIs and in particular of SMR-based BCIs is the detection of a non-intention condition, during which a user does not want to send any command. This so-called zero-class problem is often handled in brain switch implementations by defining one MI class as the resting class or to use long MIs to pause or reactivate the system.[10] However, this approach is not appropriate for all applications, which renders the zero-class problem as one of the major limiting factors for the practical use of SMR-BCIs.

Hybrid BCIs

A novel development in noninvasive BCI research is the introduction of the hybrid BCI (hBCI) concept.[11] An hBCI consists of a combination of multiple BCIs or a BCI with other input devices. These input devices may be based on the registration of biosignals other than brain signals, such as myoelectric activities. The hBCI concept helps to overcome limitations inherent to a singular BCI system, such as false-positive, unintended decisions or the zero-class problem. In fact, the second input signal can be effectively used to indicate an "idling" state or to introduce a context-specific correction mechanism. Using this approach, a user can generate a single command signal either by fusing different input signals or by simply selecting one of them. In the latter situation, the input signals must not be static, but can be dynamically routed based on their reliability. In the case of signal fusion, each of the input signals contributes to the overall command signal with a dedicated weighting factor, which can also be dynamically adjusted.

An example for demonstration of the superiority of this approach is an hBCI-controlled telepresence robot that the user navigates to the left and right by imagination of movements of the left and right hand and stops/starts the movements of the robot by an electromyographic switch activated by a short muscle twitch. In an hBCI-controlled communication application based on two BCIs (P300 and SSVEP), SSVEP activity is used to assess whether the subject is focused on a spelling task. If no SSVEP activity is found, then the system assumes that the user is not paying attention to the spelling system and does not output any characters. Another example is an hBCI-controlled reaching and grasping neuroprosthesis, in which the hBCI consists of an SMR-BCI combined with an analog shoulder joystick.[9] The neuroprosthesis is activated/deactivated by a long MI detected by the SMR-BCI. Short MIs switch between shoulder and elbow control, while the degree of hand closing and elbow flexion is controlled by shoulder movements. This comprehensive list of examples shows that the hBCI concept is a valuable extension of established user interfaces and may allow more users to effectively control new assistive technology or may simplify the use of existing devices.

Application of BCIs in Individuals with Spinal Cord Injury

Most of the results in BCI research have been obtained with able-bodied subjects; only a few (< 5%) BCI studies involved impaired users with a real need for a BCI. BCI research in patients with SCI has been performed thus far only in individuals in the chronic stage, at the earliest 1 year after the onset of the injury in a stable neurologic, psychological, and social state.[12]

BCIs for Computer Access

The current BCIs for computer access, communication, and entertainment purposes are mostly ERP-based BCIs working with the P300

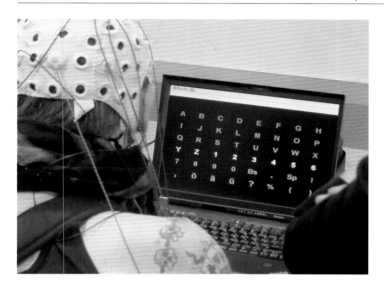

Fig. 14.1 A subject with tetraplegia using a flashing character matrix speller with a P300-based brain–computer interface (BCI).

signal. Numerous clinical studies confirm the efficacy of the P300-BCI in paralyzed patients with four choice responses, such as "Yes/No/ Pass/End" or "Up/Down/Left/Right," for cursor movement. With P300-spellers, words could be composed letter by letter, which are arranged in a matrix fashion in rows and columns (**Fig. 14.1**). One letter is selected by implementation of an oddball paradigm, in which rows and columns are highlighted randomly while the user focuses on one specific letter (target letter) that he or she wishes to select and tries to ignore all other letters that are highlighted in other rows or columns (nontarget letters). Each time the target letter is highlighted, a P300 signal occurs in the frontoparietal brain region. Each target letter can be identified by a classifier that detects the occurrence of a P300 signal every time the row and column of the intended letter is highlighted, and selects the letter accordingly. In a recent study, a new paradigm was introduced for enhancement of the P300 control, in which a famous face, in this case the face of Albert Einstein, is superimposed on top of the matrix display.[13] By the implementation of this paradigm, patients who were formerly unable to control a traditional P300-based speller were enabled to successfully use this kind of communication interface.

An alternative to P300-based spellers is SMR-based spelling systems such as the Hex-o-Spell paradigm. In this paradigm, hexagons filled with groups of letters or a single letter are arranged in a circular fashion with a pointing arrow in the center of the circle. The circle can be rotated by one type of motor imagery (e.g., right hand movements), and extended for selection with another motor imagery (e.g., foot movements).

Although the traditional matrix-based P300-based spellers are the most widespread type of BCIs used for communication purposes, alternative BCIs using different designs and signal modalities such as SSVEPs are developed to build a faster, more accurate, less mentally demanding and more satisfying BCI. Such systems may enable basic communication in individuals with very high spinal cord injury who are ventilator dependent.

■ BCIs for Wheelchair and Environmental Control

In addition to communication and manipulation, being mobile is another essential need of motor-impaired patients. Persons with severe motor disabilities are dependent on electrical wheelchairs controlled by hand- or chin-operated manual joysticks. If not enough residual movements are present, eye-gaze or suck-and-puff control units may serve as a wheelchair user interface. For suck-and-puff control, end users must be able to reliably generate two different levels of air pressure/vacuum over a sustained period of time to achieve a good level of control. Because these prerequisites are not present in all individuals with high SCI, BCIs may represent an alternative control option.

At the current state of the art, all types of noninvasive BCIs are providing only a limited command rate and are insufficient for dexterous control of complex applications. Thus, before the successful application of control interfaces with low command rates, including BCIs, in mobility devices, intelligent control schemes have to be implemented. Ideally, the user only has to issue basic navigation commands such as left, right, and forward, which are interpreted by the wheelchair controller integrating contextual information obtained from environmental sensors. Based on these interpretations, the wheelchair would perform intelligent maneuvers including obstacle avoidance and guided turnings. In such a control scheme, the responsibilities are shared between the user, who gives high-level commands, and the system, which executes low-level interactions with a greater or lesser degree of autonomy. With this so-called shared control principle, researchers have demonstrated the feasibility of mentally controlling complex mobility devices by noninvasive BCIs, despite its slow information transfer rate.[12]

Another important goal is to enable severely paralyzed patients to control their environment independently, to which BCIs may contribute significantly. First results in users with handicaps show that environmental control by an asynchronous P300 BCI is possible. However, system testing also demonstrated that the minimum number of stimulation sequences needed for correct classification had a higher intrasubject variability in users with respect to what was previously observed in young, non-disabled controls.[14] Also, special focus must be

put on the design of the visual control interface to achieve high accuracy while keeping mental effort low.

BCIs for Control of Robotic Lower Extremity Exoskeletons

Motorized lower extremity exoskeletons are an emerging technology. They have recently become commercially available for clinical and personal use. Although devices from different manufacturers vary substantially in their technical specifications and intended field of application, their common goal is to compensate for a lost standing and walking function. Potential users need to fulfill many prerequisites, such as sufficient trunk stability and minimal spasticity/joint contractures, to successfully use these systems in everyday life. But as technology progresses, the combination of an exoskeleton and a SMR-based BCI able to detect the user's intention to walk hold promise to technically bridge the injured spinal cord. First implementations show the feasibility of such an approach.[15]

BCIs for Control of an Upper Extremity Neuroprosthesis

Neuroprostheses based on functional electrical stimulation (FES) represent the only possibility for at least partial restoration of permanently restricted or lost functions in case of missing surgical options. Over the last three decades, FES systems with different levels of complexity were developed, and some of them were successfully transferred into clinical routine. FES systems deliver short current impulses eliciting physiological action potentials on efferent nerves, which cause contractions of the innervated but paralyzed muscles of the arm. On this basis, FES artificially compensates for the loss of voluntary muscle control. The simplest form of a neuroprosthesis is based on the application of multiple surface electrodes. With only seven surface electrodes placed on the forearm, which is a small number, two grasp patterns, namely a key grasp and power grasp, can be restored.[16]

Through the last decade, it has become obvious that the user interface of all current FES devices is not optimal for providing natural control. In the case of individuals with a high, complete SCI and the associated severe disabilities, not enough residual functions are preserved for control in the form of either movements or underlying muscle activation from a nonparalyzed body part. This has been a major limitation in the development of a reaching neuroprostheses for individuals with a loss not only of hand and finger function but also of elbow and shoulder function.

In 2003, a pioneering work showed for the first time that a MI-BCI control of a neuroprosthesis based on surface electrodes is feasible.[17] In this single case study, the restoration of a lateral grasp was achieved in a tetraplegic patient who suffers from a chronic SCI with completely missing hand and finger function. The patient was able to move through a predefined sequence of grasp phases by imagination of foot movements detected by an SMR-BCI with 100% accuracy. He reached this performance level prior to the experiment by undergoing several weeks of training with the MI-BCI, and he has maintained it for almost a decade by participating in periodic continuing-training sessions.[18]

A second feasibility experiment has been performed, in which a short-term BCI training program was applied in another individual with tetraplegia. This subject was using a Freehand system for several years. After 3 days of training, he was able to control the grasp sequence of the implanted neuroprosthesis with a moderate, but sufficient performance.[19]

In these first attempts, the BCI was used as a substitute for the traditional neuroprosthesis control interface rather than as an extension. With the introduction of FES-hybrid orthoses, it becomes more important to increase the number of independent control signals. With the recent implementation of the hBCI framework, it became feasible to use a combination of input signals rather than BCI alone. In a first single case study, a combination of a MI-BCI and an analog shoulder position sensor is proposed. By upward/downward movements of the shoulder, the user can control the degree of elbow flexion/extension or of hand opening/closing. The routing of the analog signal from the shoulder position sensor to the control of the elbow or the hand and the access to a pause state is determined by a digital signal provided by the MI-BCI. By briefly imagining a hand movement, the user switches from hand to elbow control or vice versa. A longer activation leads to a pause state with stimulation turned off or reactivates the system from the pause state. With this setup, a highly paralyzed patient who had no preserved voluntary elbow, hand, and finger movements was able to perform several activities of daily living, among them eating a pretzel stick and an ice cone and signing a document (**Fig. 14.2**), which previously he was not able to perform without the neuroprosthesis.[16]

▓ Invasive BCIs

Although noninvasive, EEG-based BCIs are easily available and were successfully used by individuals with acute as well as chronic SCI, they present several problems: Although temporal resolution is generally good, spatial resolution of noninvasive BCIs is rather poor due to the summed recording of signals from large cell populations. The poor selectivity is the reason that, with noninvasive BCIs, an intuitive, simultaneous control of many degrees of freedom is hardly possible. The signal-to-noise ratio of EEG-based systems and the temporal resolution are limited because of the low-pass characteristics of the bony structures of the skull. Noninvasive BCIs are prone to artifacts caused by movements of electrodes and caps and by crosstalk from muscles, such as during eye movements. Most of the electrodes of BCI

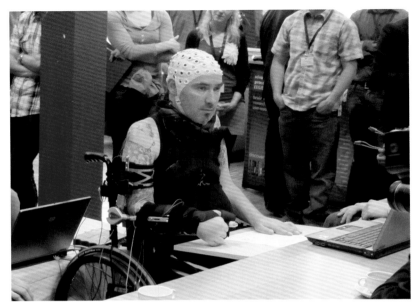

Fig. 14.2 A subject with tetraplegia and completely absent finger, hand, and elbow function using a motor imagery (MI)-BCI–controlled hybrid functional electrical stimulation (FES) elbow orthosis and a grasp neuroprosthesis to sign a document.

systems need contact gel, which results in a relatively time-consuming montage (e.g., montage of 12 Laplace electrodes needed for a typical 2-class SMR-BCI in approx. 20 minutes) and needs to be washed out of the hair after use.

Most of the disadvantages of noninvasive BCIs can be overcome by invasive BCIs, where electrodes for recording of brain activity are implanted intracranially. Although it is known that many cortical areas contribute to the planning and execution of movements, the primary motor cortex (M1) is assumed to be the area most involved in motor actions. The site of implantation can vary from extradural to intraparenchymal, depending on the technology of the electrodes. In general, invasive electrodes are directly placed onto or in the cortex, which enables the recording of multiple forms of electrical potentials such as high-frequency oscillations, local field potentials (LFPs), and spikes from single or multiple neurons. LFPs are promising sources for real-time control of multidimensional assistive devices such as robot arms, because they seem to be more robust, and the high-gamma LFP recordings may contain more information about executed or imagined movements than recordings from single neurons.

BCIs Based on Electrocorticographic Recordings

The least invasive BCI is based on the recording of the electrocorticogram (ECoG). The electrodes typically consist of platinum disks with a diameter of 2 to 3 mm embedded in a silicon or polymer sheet. These sheets are placed epi- or subdurally, but never penetrate the brain tissue and therefore entail only a low risk of damage of the neuronal tissue. With ECoG- and microECoG-based BCIs, local electrical field changes can be recorded with far better spatial resolution than with noninvasive electrical BCIs. As in EEG-based BCIs, the modulation of cortical activity patterns is robust and stable once they have been established by training. It recently has been shown in an individual with an SCI at the level of C4 that a three-dimensional (3D) cursor control can be achieved within a training period of about 20 days.[20] In this case, the grid was removed according to the study protocol after 28 days, which unfortunately makes it impossible to evaluate the BCI performance and the stability of the brain signals over a longer period of time. The few observations that were made with long-term implantations of ECoG electrode grids indicate that the limited fluid exchange and the mechanical irritation of the brain tissue by the rigid electrode grid lead to signs of chronic inflammation. However, this may be prevented by the future development of very thin, flexible, and porous grids. For minimization of the risk of infections including wound infections, meningitis, and osteomyelitis due to the transcutaneous wires, a fully implantable ECoG grid would be highly desirable but is not yet available for human use. Surgery-related and noninfectious complications, among them cerebrospinal fluid leaks, neurologic injuries, and subdural/deep hemorrhage, represent a general problem in invasive BCIs, which need to be clearly communicated to users prior to implantation.[3]

▦ BCIs Based on Intracortical Recordings

The spatial resolution of ECoG recordings is still not sufficient for decoding of imagery of fine motor skills, such as movements of single finger joints. Higher spatial resolution can only be achieved with intracortical recordings. For this purpose, high-density, multichannel electrodes were developed that are implanted into the neocortex either epipial or intraparenchymal and record single-cell activities through cone electrodes or microelectrode arrays (MEAs). Most of the research performed on BCIs with intracortical recordings is based on the Utah array MEA, which is commercially available from Blackrock Microsystems (Salt Lake City, UT). This array consists of 100 needle electrodes, which are placed on a rectangular carrier with a dimension of 4 mm × 4 mm (**Fig. 14.3**). The electrode array is wired with a trans-

cutaneous connector plug that is fixed by screws with the skullcap and transmits the signals to an amplifier mounted on top of the head. Special care needs to be taken of the area around the connector to avoid local infections and more severe adverse events such as meningitis. For implantation of the MEA, special equipment in the form of a pneumatically driven insertion device and well-trained surgeons are needed to minimize brain tissue damage.

In the most recent studies involving individuals with SCI, two intracortical MEAs were implanted in the motor cortex ~ 14 mm apart in one study[21] and in the posterior parietal cortex in another study.[22] With these implants, it was shown in a woman with tetraplegia that a very sophisticated real-time control of a robot arm with seven degrees of freedom and later with ten degrees of freedom (3D translation, 3D orientation, 4D grasping, and hand shaping) was possible with minimal training over a few days.[21,23] This level of simultaneous control of multiple degrees of freedom almost immediately after the implantation has not been achieved with noninvasive MI-SMR–based BCIs so far. From a neuroscientific viewpoint it is very interesting that the algorithm for decoding of the movement intention is initially trained with the cortical activities during observation of predefined movements of the robot arm.[24]

Although the first feasibility experiments show very promising results, huge efforts are still needed to get invasive systems out of the laboratory into the home environment of end users. As with every invasive procedure, the implantation of electrodes bears some surgical risks. Long-term complications may occur such as cerebrospinal fluid leakage or infections due to the transcutaneous wires. In any case, a fully implanted recording device needs to be developed to increase the usability and lower the risk of infections. The ultrafine structures of the electrode tips are not long-term stable, and after 5 years only a few electrodes may be left for proper recording of neuronal activity.[25] The loss of signals is mainly caused by degradation of electrode materials, gliosis, or chronic inflammation. This may be overcome by coating of the electrodes with extracellular matrix or with

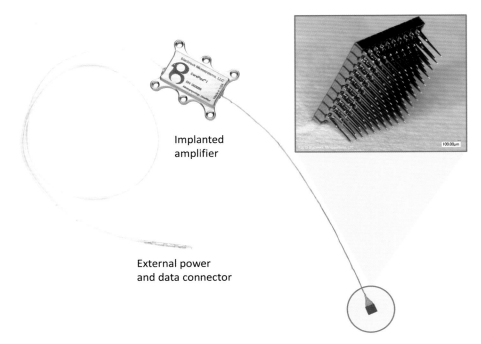

Implanted
amplifier

External power
and data connector

Fig. 14.3 The implantable Cereplex I system consisting of the Utah Array microelectrode array for intracortical recordings, an integrated amplifier and digitalization unit, and a transcutaneous lead for external energy supply and signal transmission. (Courtesy of Blackrock Microsystems, Salt Lake City, UT.)

short adherent proteins to minimize inflammatory responses and support cell proliferation and differentiation.[26] The long-term stability and biocompatibility are key prerequisites for routine clinical use of MEAs, because their removal causes additional damage to the brain tissue adhering to them. Further, it is not clear whether with a new implant the same level of performance will be reached as with the explanted device.

Although BCIs based on intracortical recordings can be operated by the user with almost no training time, daily tuning of the movement decoding algorithms is necessary. Only one third of the electrodes used for control of the robot on one day contribute to its operation on the next day. At the current state of the art, this tuning procedure needs the support of technically qualified personnel, and therefore automatic tuning algorithms need to be introduced to enable the autonomous operation of a BCI with intracortical electrodes by the users' caregivers at their homes.

▤ Future Outlook

BCIs are an evolving technology to provide people with a high SCI better control of assistive devices for a more self-determined life. Currently available BCI systems differ substantially in regard to the degree of invasiveness, the complexity of hardware and software components, the basic modes of operation, and the underlying physiological mechanisms. In recent years, noninvasive EEG-based BCIs have reached a level of maturity sufficient for home use. BCIs have been successfully used for the control of a variety of assistive devices, among them computer access and environmental control systems; wheelchairs and telepresence robots; neuroprostheses, especially of the upper extremities; and exoskeletons for the lower and upper extremities. Systems based on the MI-initiated modulation of SMRs over cortical motor areas are the preferred choice for self-paced control, in particular of devices to improve manipulation skills. With the recent introduction of hybrid BCIs combining one BCI with another or with traditional control interfaces such as eye-trackers, the number of potential BCI users is expected to increase. However, even after substantial training, not every user is able to reliably control an SMR-based BCI, and high-performing users are only able to generate a few decisions per minute. Users of noninvasive BCIs complain most about the time-consuming setup of the system, in particular of the gel electrodes. This might be overcome in the future by recently introduced wireless BCI systems based on dry or semi-dry electrodes.[27] Also the cosmetic appearance of these customizable novel systems is much better than that of the traditionally used standard EEG caps.

Although considerable progress has been made in noninvasive BCIs over the last decade, it is mainly digital control signals in the form of brain switches that can be generated. This might not be sufficient for everyday operation of complex devices such as neuroprostheses. An intuitive, simultaneous control of the multiple degrees of freedom of arm and grasp neuroprostheses or multi-joint robot arms in real time was recently shown in single-case studies using invasive BCIs based on ECoG recordings or high-density intracortical electrode arrays. Although invasive systems provide a better spatial and—to some parts—temporal resolution and a higher signal-to-noise ratio, they are associated with surgical risks and have only a limited long-term stability. Furthermore, daily tuning of the movement decoder algorithms by technical experts is necessary. These disadvantages need to be clearly communicated to potential users, who at the current state of the art seem to prefer noninvasive solutions.[3] This may change in the future, if intracortical electrode arrays will not only be used for the detection of the movement intention, but also provide sensory feedback by stimulation of cortical sensory neurons. Then the vision of a true bidirectional neuroprosthesis will become reality, representing a technical bypass around the injury of the spinal cord.[28]

Invasive and noninvasive BCIs are companions rather than competitors, because some users will not agree to undergo surgery in their unaffected brain and others are not willing to

undergo a substantial period of training for only a few degrees of control. Although BCIs are a promising technology for user interfaces in individuals with high cervical lesions, more clinical trials involving a larger number of impaired users are needed to obtain objective information about the users' satisfaction and increased quality of life. In invasive BCIs, the long-term risk/benefit ratio needs to be evaluated.

Up to now, the focus of the application of BCIs mainly lies in their use as an assistive devices control interface for substitution of lost function in chronic SCI. However, BCIs for detection of motor imagery offer further possibilities in the context of the rehabilitation of patients with acute or subacute SCI that goes beyond the control of assistive device. After an SCI, substantial reorganization of neural networks occurs in brain and spinal cord that plays a critical role for functional recovery and may be the origin of secondary lesion-associated complications like neuropathic pain. The basis for the therapeutic use of BCIs is that the central nervous system shows a lifelong ability for neural plasticity, which can be enhanced after a trauma or injury by task-specific training. The key elements for an effective neurorehabilitative training based on motor learning are voluntarily generated movement intentions and a synchronized sensory and proprioceptive feedback of the limbs' motor actions.[29] BCIs hold promise to enable the detection of intended movements, for example of the hand, even in patients with high SCI, making them an ideal tool for closed-loop neurorehabilitative therapies when used in combination with a grasping and reaching neuroprosthesis.[30] Additionally, by practicing feedback-controlled MI of paralyzed limbs, the integrity of cortical neuronal connections may be preserved or neurologic recovery of motor function may be even enhanced. The latter goal has already been demonstrated in the rehabilitation of upper extremity motor functions in stroke survivors.[31] The potential of BCIs for compensation or substitution of a lost function and restoration of a restricted function after SCI has not yet been fully exploited, and further fields of application of the BCI technology will develop in the future.

■ Chapter Summary

People with high cervical SCIs are in great need of assistive technology to provide electronic media access, environmental control, and substitution of lost manipulation capabilities. But options for user interfaces are very limited in patients with severe motor impairments.

Brain–computer interfaces are devices that measure brain activities and translate them into control signals. Current implementations of BCIs differ substantially in regard to the degree of invasiveness, the complexity of hardware and software components, the basic modes of operation, and the underlying physiological mechanisms. In recent years, noninvasive BCIs based on EEG recordings have reached a level of maturity sufficient for home use.

The controlled applications of BCIs range from computer access and environmental control systems, to wheelchairs and telepresence robots, to neuroprostheses and exoskeletons. Systems based on the modulation of SMRs by motor imagery are the preferred choice for self-paced control. With the recent introduction of hybrid BCIs, combining one BCI with another or with traditional control interfaces, the number of potential BCI users is expected to increase. However, even after substantial training, not every user is able to reliably control an SMR-based BCI, and high-performing users are only able to generate a few decisions per minute.

An intuitive control of arm and grasp neuroprostheses or multi-joint robot arms is currently only achievable with invasive BCIs based on the recording of the ECoG or high-density intracortical electrode arrays. Although invasive systems provide better spatial and temporal resolution and a higher signal-to-noise ratio, they are associated with surgical risks and have a limited long-term stability. Furthermore, daily tuning of the movement decoding algorithms by technical experts is necessary.

Although BCIs are a promising technology for individuals with SCI, more clinical trials are needed for assessment of users' satisfaction and increased quality of life.

Pearls

◆ Brain–computer interfaces are an evolving technology for enhancement of the control of assistive devices for communication/entertainment, mobility, and manipulation in patients with a high cervical SCI.
◆ In recent years, noninvasive EEG-based BCIs reached a level of maturity in hardware and software that is sufficient for home use.
◆ In the research setting with invasive BCIs, a decoding of imagined movements is possible sufficient for real-time control of multi-joint robot arms.
◆ Hybrid-BCIs as a combination of one BCI with another or with established user interfaces increase the number of potential users.

Pitfalls

◆ One has to be aware that BCI is a rather general term used for systems with very different degrees of invasiveness, underlying physiological mechanisms, and signal analysis algorithms.
◆ In noninvasive BCIs, not every user may achieve a level of performance sufficient for control (hence the term "BCI-illiteracy").
◆ In invasive BCIs, surgical risks needs to be considered and clearly communicated to potential users.
◆ Intracortical BCIs have to be recalibrated on a daily basis for proper operation, which at the current state of the art needs highly qualified technical support.
◆ More clinical studies are needed to identify the benefit of BCIs in the rehabilitation of acute patients and the impact on quality of life in users with chronic SCI.

References

Five Must-Read References
1. National Spinal Cord Injury Statistical Center. The 2014 annual statistical report for the model spinal cord injury care system. https://www.nscisc.uab.edu/PublicDocuments/reports/pdf/2014%20NSCISC%20Annual%20Statistical%20Report%20Complete%20Public%20Version.pdf. Accessed August 3, 2015
2. Zickler C, Donna VD, Kaiser V, et al. BCI-Applications for People with Disabilities: Defining User Needs and User Requirements. Assistive Technology from Adapted Equipment to Inclusive Environments: AAATE. Amsterdam: IOS Press; 2009:185–189
3. Blabe CH, Gilja V, Chestek CA, Shenoy KV, Anderson KD, Henderson JM. Assessment of brain-machine

interfaces from the perspective of people with paralysis. J Neural Eng 2015;12:043002

4. Wolpaw JR, Birbaumer N, McFarland DJ, Pfurtscheller G, Vaughan TM. Brain-computer interfaces for communication and control. Clin Neurophysiol 2002; 113:767–791

5. Nicolas-Alonso LF, Gomez-Gil J. Brain computer interfaces, a review. Sensors (Basel) 2012;12:1211–1279

6. Kleih SC, Kaufmann T, Zickler C, et al. Out of the frying pan into the fire—the P300-based BCI faces real-world challenges. Prog Brain Res 2011;194: 27–46

7. Kaiser V, Bauernfeind G, Kreilinger A, et al. Cortical effects of user training in a motor imagery based brain-computer interface measured by fNIRS and EEG. Neuroimage 2014;85(Pt 1):432–444

8. McFarland DJ, Sarnacki WA, Wolpaw JR. Electroencephalographic (EEG) control of three-dimensional movement. J Neural Eng 2010;7:036007

9. Rohm M, Schneiders M, Müller C, et al. Hybrid brain-computer interfaces and hybrid neuroprostheses for restoration of upper limb functions in individuals with high-level spinal cord injury. Artif Intell Med 2013;59:133–142

10. Rupp R. Challenges in clinical applications of brain computer interfaces in individuals with spinal cord injury. Front Neuroeng 2014;7:38

11. Müller-Putz G, Leeb R, Tangermann M, et al. Towards noninvasive hybrid brain-computer interfaces: framework, practice, clinical application, and beyond. P IEEE 2015;103:926–943

12. Millán JD, Rupp R, Müller-Putz GR, et al. Combining brain-computer interfaces and assistive technologies: state-of-the-art and challenges. Front Neurosci 2010;4:161

13. Kaufmann T, Schulz SM, Koblitz A, Renner G, Wessig C, Kübler A. Face stimuli effectively prevent brain-computer interface inefficiency in patients with neurodegenerative disease. Clin Neurophysiol 2012

14. Aloise F, Schettini F, Aricò P, et al. Asynchronous P300-based brain-computer interface to control a virtual environment: initial tests on end users. Clin EEG Neurosci 2011;42:219–224

15. Contreras-Vidal J, Presacco A, Agashe H, Paek A. Restoration of whole body movement: toward a noninvasive brain-machine interface system. IEEE Pulse 2012;3:34–37

16. Rupp R, Rohm M, Schneiders M, Kreilinger A, Müller-Putz GR. Functional rehabilitation of the paralyzed upper extremity after spinal cord injury by noninvasive hybrid neuroprostheses. Proc IEEE. 2015;103: 954–968

17. Pfurtscheller G, Müller GR, Pfurtscheller J, Gerner HJ, Rupp R. "Thought"-control of functional electrical stimulation to restore hand grasp in a patient with tetraplegia. Neurosci Lett 2003;351:33–36

18. Enzinger C, Ropele S, Fazekas F, et al. Brain motor system function in a patient with complete spinal cord injury following extensive brain-computer interface training. Exp Brain Res 2008;190:215–223

19. Müller-Putz GR, Scherer R, Pfurtscheller G, Rupp R. EEG-based neuroprosthesis control: a step towards clinical practice. Neurosci Lett 2005;382:169–174

20. Wang W, Collinger JL, Degenhart AD, et al. An electrocorticographic brain interface in an individual with tetraplegia. PLoS ONE 2013;8:e55344

21. Collinger JL, Wodlinger B, Downey JE, et al. High-performance neuroprosthetic control by an individual with tetraplegia. Lancet 2013;381:557–564

22. Aflalo T, Kellis S, Klaes C, et al. Neurophysiology. Decoding motor imagery from the posterior parietal cortex of a tetraplegic human. Science 2015;348: 906–910

23. Wodlinger B, Downey JE, Tyler-Kabara EC, Schwartz AB, Boninger ML, Collinger JL. Ten-dimensional anthropomorphic arm control in a human brain-machine interface: difficulties, solutions, and limitations. J Neural Eng 2015;12:016011

24. Hiremath SV, Chen W, Wang W, et al. Brain computer interface learning for systems based on electrocorticography and intracortical microelectrode arrays. Front Integr Nuerosci 2015;9:40

25. Hochberg LR, Bacher D, Jarosiewicz B, et al. Reach and grasp by people with tetraplegia using a neurally controlled robotic arm. Nature 2012;485:372–375

26. Gunasekera B, Saxena T, Bellamkonda R, Karumbaiah L. Intracortical recording interfaces: current challenges to chronic recording function. ACS Chem Neurosci 2015;6:68–83

27. Lee S, Shin S, Woo S, Kim K, Lee H-N. Review of wireless brain-computer interface systems. In: Fazel-Rezai R, ed. Brain-Computer Interface Systems—Recent Progress and Future Prospects, Intech, Rijeka, Croatia. 2013

28. Collinger JL, Foldes S, Bruns TM, Wodlinger B, Gaunt R, Weber DJ. Neuroprosthetic technology for individuals with spinal cord injury. J Spinal Cord Med 2013;36:258–272

29. Jackson A, Zimmermann JB. Neural interfaces for the brain and spinal cord—restoring motor function. Nat Rev Neurol 2012;8:690–699

30. Tidoni E, Tieri G, Aglioti SM. Re-establishing the disrupted sensorimotor loop in deafferented and deefferented people: The case of spinal cord injuries. Neuropsychologia 2015;79(Pt B):301–309

31. Pichiorri F, Morone G, Petti M, et al. Brain-computer interface boosts motor imagery practice during stroke recovery. Ann Neurol 2015;77:851–865

Index

Note: Page references followed by *f* or *t* indicate figures or tables, respectively

A

ActiGraph wGT3X-BT device, 174–175, 175f
Action potentials, 148–149
Activity monitoring devices, 174–175, 175f
Advanced Trauma Life Support (ATLS) protocol, 57–58
Agarose, 108t, 113–114
Airway management, 57–58
Alginate, 108t, 114–115
Ambulation. *See* Walking
American Association of Neurological Surgeons (AANS)/Congress of Neurological Surgeons (CNS), 95–97
American Spinal Injury Association (ASIA)
  Impairment Scale (AIS), 14, 14t, 25–26, 37
    "ceiling effect," 37–38
    of early surgical decompression effects, 73, 74f, 95
    International SCI Data Sets, 21–22
    International Standards for Neurological Classification of Spinal Cord Injury (ISNCSI), 13–16, 15f, 22, 25, 35, 41
Amyotrophic lateral sclerosis patients, brain-computer interface technology for, 157
Antibodies, for masking extracellular inhibitory molecules, 137–138, 145
Antibody-based immunomodulation, neuroprotective effects of, 102
Antioxidants, 3–4
Apoptosis, 6, 57
Aretech ZeroG®, 164–166, 166f
Armeo® Spring, 173–174, 173f
Assistive technology, 21
  brain-computer interfaces for, 179–191
    application of, 182
    for communication, 157, 182–183, 183f

    components of, 179–180
    for computer access, 182–183, 183f
    definition of, 179, 190
    electrocorticographic recordings (ECoG)-based, 157, 186–187, 189, 190
    electroencephalogram (EEG)-based, 157, 180, 180t, 185–186, 187
    for environmental control, 184
    event-related potential (ERP)-based, 180–181, 182–183
    functional electrical stimulation (FES)-based, 156–159, 159f, 160f
    future outlook for, 188–189
    hybrid, 182, 188–189, 190
    invasive devices, 185–188, 189, 190
    mechanism of, 156–157
    in movement facilitation technologies, 158–159
    for neurorehabilitation, 157
    noninvasive, 179–185, 188–189, 190
    for robotic lower extremity exoskeleton control, 157, 184
    sensorimotor rhythm (SRM)-based, 181–182, 184, 188–189
    steady-state evoked potential (SSEP)-based, 181
    for upper extremity neuroprothesis control, 157, 184–185, 186f
    for wheelchair control, 157, 183–184
  for gait training, 164–168, 165f, 166f, 170, 172, 176
Astrocytes, in spinal cord injury, 90f–91f
Autonomic dysfunction, spinal cord injury-related, 72
  blood pressure augmentation for, 93t, 95–96
Autonomic Function after Spinal Cord Injury (ISAFSCI), 16

Axonal regeneration, in the injured spinal cord, 6–7,
132
axon growth-promoting molecules in, 107
growth inhibitors of, 132–147
extracellular matrix-associated inhibitory
molecules, 133*f*, 135–137, 136*f*–137*f*
masking or blocking of, 136*f*–137*f*, 137–139
myelin-associated inhibitory molecules, 133*f*,
134–135, 136–137*f*, 145
preventing downstream signaling of, 136*f*–137*f*,
139–140
reducing synthesis of, 136*f*–137*f*, 142–143
removal of, 140–142
hydrogel biomaterials for, 107–121

B
Balance
assistive robotic devices for, 164–166, 166*f*
functional assessment of, 18
Barthel Index (BI), 16–17
Beck Depression Inventory (BDI), 20
Berg Balance Scale (BBS), 18
Biomarkers, of spinal cord functional recovery,
25–38
definition of, 26
future directions for, 37
neuroinflammatory biomarkers, 29*t*–30*t*, 33–34,
37
structural biomarkers, 27–33, 28*t*–29*t*, 28*t*–30*t*,
36*t*, 37
Blood pressure augmentation, 93*t*, 95–96, 98–99
Blood-spinal cord barrier, in spinal cord injury, 3,
5, 7
Brain-computer interfaces, for assistive devices.
See Assistive technology, brain-computer
interfaces for
Brain-derived neurotrophic factor (BDNF), 103–104,
114
Buckminsterfullerene C60 particles, 103

C
Capabilities of Upper Extremity (CUE), 18
Cardiopulmonary management, of acute spinal cord
injury, 58–59, 60*t*
Cell death, spinal cord injury-related, 6
Cell transplantation therapy. *See* Neural stem
cell-based therapies
Center for Epidemiologic Studies Depression Scale
(CES-D), 20
Central cord syndrome, 2, 61*t*
surgical intervention for, 74–75
Central nervous system, limited regenerative
capacity of, 6–7
Cerebrospinal fluid biomarkers, for functional
recovery prediction, 26–38
neuroinflammatory biomarkers, 29*f*–30*t*,
33–34, 37
structural biomarkers, 27–33, 28*t*–29*t*, 36*t*,
37

Cerebrospinal fluid drainage, neuroprotective effects
of, 98–99, 104
Cervical collars, 2, 9
Cervical facet dislocation, surgical decompression
of, 75, 76*f*, 77, 78
Cervical spine, clinical clearance of, 44
Cervical spine injury, early surgical decompression
of, 73
Cethrin, neuroprotective effects of, 94*t*, 98, 104, 145
Children, spinal cord injury management in,
61*t*–62*t*
Chitosan, 109*t*, 115
Chondroitinase ABC, 140–142, 145
Chondroitin sulfate proteoglycans, 8, 116
Clinical initiatives, in spinal cord medicine, 12–16
Clinical trials
of methylprednisolone sodium succinate, 81–83,
87, 96–97
of neural stem cell-based therapies, 128–129, 130
neurologic assessment in, 25
of neuroprotective strategies, 89, 93*f*–94*f*, 95–102
Cochrane Review, of methylprednisolone therapy,
83, 84*f*, 87
Collagen-based hydrogels, 109*t*, 115–116
Communication, brain-computer interfaces for, 157,
182–183, 183*f*
Computed tomography (CT)
in children, 61*t*–62*t*
role in trauma protocols, 40
of spinal cord injury, 41
Computer access, brain-computer interfaces for,
182–183, 183*f*
Conservative or Early Surgical Management of
Incomplete Cervical Cord Syndrome Without
Spinal Instability (COSMIC), 75
Construct validity, of outcome measures, 12
Craig Handicap Assessment and Reporting Tech-
nique (CHART), 20–21
Criterion validity, of outcome measures, 12
Curcumin, neuroprotective effects of, 103
Cytokines, spinal cord injury-related release of, 5

D
Decompression, surgical
magnetic resonance imaging-based, 43, 54
as neuroprotective strategy, 93*t*, 95
timing of, 71–79, 72*f*, 74*f*, 76*f*
in central cord syndrome, 74–75
in cervical facet dislocation, 75, 76*f*, 77, 78
clinical evidence regarding, 73–74
in polytrauma, 75–78
preclinical evidence regarding, 73
Surgical Timing in Acute Spinal Cord Injury
Study (STASCIS), 73, 80, 83, 85, 85*t*, 95
Demyelination, spinal cord injury-related, 6
Depression, assessment of, 20
Disk herniation, imaging of, 43
Dopamine, 59
Drug delivery devices, hydrogels as, 107

E

Edema, spinal cord injury-related, 90f–91f, 104
  as functional recovery indicator, 44, 45t, 46–48
Ekso™, 170
Electrocorticography (ECoG)-based brain-computer
    interfaces, 157, 186–187, 189, 190
Electroencephalography (EEG)-based brain-
    computer interfaces, 157, 180, 180t, 185–186,
    187
Environmental control, brain-computer interfaces
    for, 184
Epidural stimulation, of the spinal cord, 152
European Multicenter Study on Human Spinal Cord
    Injury (EMSCI), 16
Event-related potential (ERP)-based brain-computer
    interfaces, 180–181, 182–183
Exo-H2 exoskeleton device, 172
Exoskeleton devices
  brain-computer interfaces for, 184, 190
  lower-extremity, 167–172, 176, 184
  upper-extremity, 167–168, 172–174, 173f
Expert panels, in spinal cord medicine, 12–16
Extracellular matrix-associated inhibitory mole-
    cules, 133f, 135–137, 136f–137f
  masking or blocking of, 136f–137f, 137–139
  preventing downstream signaling by, 136f–137f,
    139–140
  reducing synthesis of, 136f–137f, 142–143
  removal of, 140–142

F

Facet dislocation, cervical, surgical decompression
    of, 75, 76f
Face validity, of outcome measures, 12
Fibrin glues, 109t, 115
Fibroblast growth factor, neuroprotective effects of,
    99
Free radicals, 3–4, 9, 57
Functional electrical stimulation (FES), 148–162
  components of, 149–150
  definition of, 149
  orthotic/neuroprosthetic applications of,
    150–154, 184–185
    for reaching and grasping, 152–154, 153f
    for standing, 150
    for walking, 150–152, 151f
  therapeutic applications of, 150, 154–160
    brain-computer interfacing-controlled,
      156–159, 159f, 160f
    future directions for, 156–157
    mechanisms of recovery in, 155–156, 161
    for walking, 154–155
Functional Independence Measure (FIM), 17, 18, 47
  applied to methylprednisolone clinical trials, 82
Functional status assessment, in spinal cord injury,
    11–24. See also Outcome measures, for spinal
    cord injury
  in acute spinal cord injury, 59t
  of autonomic function, 16

of general functional status, 16–17
International Classification of Functioning,
    Disability and Health (ICF), 12
of neurologic function, 16

G

Gacyclidine, neuroprotective effects of, 101
Gait training, assistive technology for, 164–168,
    165f, 166f, 170, 172, 176
Glial fibrillary acidic protein (GFAP), as spinal cord
    injury biomarker, 27, 28t, 37
Glial scarring, 7–8, 57, 133f
Glutamate excitotoxicity, spinal cord injury-related,
    4, 9, 72
GM_1-gangliosides
  contraindications to, 61t
  neuroprotective effects of, 80, 94t, 101–102
Graded Redefined Assessment of Strength, Sen-
    sibility, and Prehension (GRASSP), 19
Granulocyte colony-stimulating factor, neuro-
    protective effects of, 100, 104
Grasp and Release Test (GRT), 18
Grasping
  assistive technology for, 152–154, 153f, 157,
    160f
  functional assessment of, 18, 19
Growth factors, neuroprotective effects of, 99, 104
Growth inhibitors, of spinal cord injury repair,
    132–147
  extracellular matrix-associated inhibitory
    molecules, 133f, 135–137, 136f–137f
  masking or blocking of, 136f–137f, 137–139
  myelin-associated inhibitory molecules, 7, 8, 8f,
    9, 133f, 134–135, 136f–137f, 145
  preventing downstream signaling of, 136f–137f,
    139–140
  reducing synthesis of, 136f–137f, 142–143
  removal of, 140–142

H

HAL exoskeleton device, 172
Hemorrhage, spinal cord injury-related, 72, 90f–91f,
    104
  intramedullary, as functional recovery indicator,
    44, 45t, 46–47, 48f
Hepatocyte growth factor, neuroprotective effects
    of, 99
Hoover's sign, 58
Hyaluronic acid, 109t, 117
Hydrogel biomaterials, for spinal cord repair and
    regeneration, 107–121
  as drug delivery devices, 107
  natural polymer-derived, 108t–109t, 113–117,
    118
  properties of, 107–118, 108t–109t, 110f
  synthetic polymer-derived, 108t, 111–113, 118
Hyperbaric oxygen therapy, 99–100
Hypotension, spinal cord injury-related, 93t, 95–96
Hypothermia, therapeutic, 80, 97, 104

I

Immobilization, of spinal cord injury patients, 58, 59*t*
  cervical collars, 2, 9
Indego®, 170–171, 171*f*
Inflammatory cascade, 102
InMotion ARM™ Robot, 172–173
Interleukins
  antibody-based immunomodulation of, 102
  as spinal cord injury biomarkers, 26, 33–34
International Campaign for Cures of Spinal Cord Injury Paralysis (ICCP), 13, 21
International Classification of Functioning, Disability and Health (ICF), 12
International SCI Data Sets, 21–22
International Spinal Cord Injury Basic Pain Database (ISCIPDS:B), 19–20
International Spinal Cord Injury Pain (ISCIP) Classification, 19, 19*t*
International Spinal Cord Society (ISCoS), 16, 21–22
International Spinal Research Trust (ISRT), 48
International Standards for Neurological Classification of Spinal Cord Injury (ISNCSCI), 13–16, 15*f*, 22, 25, 35, 41
  limitations in, 25
Intracortical recordings-based brain-computer interfaces, 187–188, 188*f*
Intravenous immunoglobulin G, 102, 104
Intubation, in acute spinal cord injury patients, 58
Ionic dysregulation, spinal cord injury-related, 4, 9, 72
Ischemia, spinal cord injury-related, 3, 9, 22, 43, 72, 104

L

Lecithinized superoxide dismutase, 103
Leeds Assessment of Neuropathic Symptoms and Signs (LANSS), 19
Life Satisfaction Questionnaires (LISAT), 20
Ligamentous injuries, magnetic resonance imaging of, 40, 43–44, 54
Lipid peroxidation, 57
Lokomat®, 164, 165*f*
Lower extremity, exoskeleton devices for, 167–172, 176, 184
LOwer extremity Powered ExoSkeleton (LOPES), 167–168
Lymphocytes, in spinal cord injury, 6

M

Macrophages, in spinal cord injury, 5–6, 90*f*–91*f*, 104
Magnesium, neuroprotective effects of, 101
Magnetic resonance angiography, of vertebral artery injuries, 40, 44, 54
Magnetic resonance imaging, of the injured spinal cord, 39–56
  advanced techniques in, 48–54, 50*t*, 55
  advantages and disadvantages of, 40–41, 55

  for cervical spine clinical clearance, 44
  conventional MRI, 40–54
  future directions in, 54
  gradient echo imaging, 42, 42*t*
  ligamentous injury, 40, 43–44, 54
  prior to facet dislocation reduction, 75, 77, 78
  short-tau inversion recovery (STIR) sequence, 42, 42*t*
  of spinal cord compression, 40, 42–43, 54
  susceptibility weighted imaging, 42
  T1-weighted imaging, 41–42, 42*t*
  T2-weighted imaging, 41, 42*t*
  trauma protocols for, 40–41
  of vertebral artery injuries, 40, 44, 54
Matrigel, 109*t*, 117
Maximum canal compromise (MCC), 44, 45*t*, 46*f*, 47
Maximum spinal cord compression (MSCC), 44, 45*t*, 46*f*
Mean arterial pressure (MAP) elevation, for hypotension management, 93*t*, 95–96, 98–99, 104
Methylprednisolone sodium succinate (MPSS), as acute spinal cord injury treatment
  contraindication to, 61*t*, 96
  evidence for, 81–85, 84*f*, 85*t*, 86, 87
    clinical trials, 81–83, 87, 96–97
    preclinical studies, 81–82, 96
  neuroprotective effects of, 93*t*, 96–97
  practice guidelines for, 85–87, 96–97
Microelectrode arrays, for brain-computer interfaces, 187–188, 188*f*
Microglia, in spinal cord injury, 90*f*–91*f*, 104
MicroRNA, as spinal cord injury biomarker, 30*t*, 34–35
Microtuble-associated protein-2 (MAP-2), as spinal cord injury biomarker, 27, 28*t*, 31, 37
Minocycline, neuroprotective effects of, 80, 93*t*, 98, 104
Mitochondrial dysfunction, 4, 57
Modified Ashworth Scale (MAS), 21
Modified Barthel Index (MBI), 16–17
Monocyte chemoattractant protein-1 (MCP-1), as spinal cord injury biomarker, 30*t*, 34, 37
Motor examination, 41
Movement facilitation technologies, 148–149, 158–159, 159*f*
Myelin-associated inhibitory molecules, 7, 8, 8*f*, 9, 133*f*, 134–135, 136*f*–137*f*, 145
  masking or blocking of, 136*f*–137*f*, 137–139
  preventing downstream signaling by, 136*f*–137*f*, 139–140
  reducing synthesis of, 136*f*–137*f*, 142–143
  removal of, 140–142

N

Naloxone, neuroprotective effects of, 80, 93*t*, 101
Nanoparticles, neuroprotective effects of, 102–103, 104

National Acute Spinal Cord Injury Study I (NASCIS I), 81, 87, 96
National Acute Spinal Cord Injury Study II (NASCIS II), 81–83, 87, 96
National Acute Spinal Cord Injury Study III (NASCIS III), 81, 82, 87
Necrosis, spinal cord injury-related, 6, 57, 90f–91f
Neural stem cell-based therapies, for spinal cord repair, 122–131
    cellular sources for, 126–128, 127f
    clinical trials of, 128–129, 130
    neuronal relay concept of, 125–126
    rationales for, 124
    robustness of therapeutic effect of, 124–125
    underlying mechanisms of, 124
Neurofilaments, as spinal cord injury biomarkers, 28t–29t, 31, 37
Neuroimaging, 16. *See also* Computed tomography; Magnetic resonance imaging; X-rays
Neuroinflammation, spinal cord injury-related, 5
Neurologic deficits
    assessment of, 25–26, 35, 37, 41, 59t
    rostral to C4, 179
Neurologic outcomes
    biomarkers for, 25–38
    effect of surgical intervention timing on, 71–79, 72f, 74f
    factors affecting, 57
    magnetic resonance imaging-based prediction of, 44–48, 45t, 55
    measures of, 16
Neuromuscular electrical stimulation (NES), 149
Neuronal relay concept, of neural stem cell-based therapy, 125–126
Neuron-specific enolase, as spinal cord injury biomarker, 31–32, 37
Neuroprotective strategies, for the injured spinal cord, 89–106
    clinical trials of, 89, 93f–94f, 95–102
    pathophysiological basis for, 89, 90f–92f
    preclinical studies of, 102–104
Neuroprotheses. *See also* Assistive technology
    brain-computer interfaces for, 157, 184–185, 186f, 190
    definition of, 149
    for standing, 150
    for walking, 150–152, 151f, 157
Nimodipine, neuroprotective effects of, 80, 94t, 101
Nogo, 7, 8f, 9
Nogo-A, 136f–137f, 138–139
Numerical Rating Scale (NRS), for pain assessment, 19
Nutritional support, 63t

O
Oligodendrocyte precursor cells, in spinal cord injury, 91f
Oligodendrocytes, in spinal cord injury, 6, 7, 8, 90f–91f

Outcome measures, for spinal cord injury, 11–24
    for assistive technology use, 21
    of autonomic function, 16
    clinical initiatives in, 12–16, 14t, 15f
    for depression, 20
    face validity of, 12
    of general functional status, 16–17, 22
    of neurologic function, 16
    for nontraumatic spinal cord injuries, 22
    for pain, 19–20, 19t
    quality of, 11–12
    for quality of life, 20–21
    recent psychometric parameters for, 22
    reliability of, 11–12
    for spasticity, 21
    of upper extremity function, 18–19, 22
    validity of, 11–12
    of walking, ambulation, and balance, 17–18, 22
Outcome Measures Toolkit, 13
Outcomes, for spinal cord injury, magnetic resonance imaging-based prediction of, 44–48, 46f, 48f, 55

P
Pain, assessment and classification of, 19–20, 19t, 60t
PAM/POGO gait training device, 168
Patient Health Questionnaire-9 (PHQ-9), 20
Penn Spasm Frequency Scale (PSFS), 21
Peripheral nervous system, injury repair in, 132, 144–145
Phenylephrine, 59
Phrenic nerve injury, 58
Poly(2-hydroxyethyl methacrylate) (pHEMA), 108t, 112
Poly(2-hydroxypropyl methacrylamide) (pHPMA), 108t, 112
Polyethylene glycol (PEG), 108t, 111–112
Polylactic acid (PLA), 108t, 112–113
Polylactic-Co-glycolic acid (PLGA), 108t, 112–113
Polytrauma patients, surgical decompression in, 75–78
Progenitor cells, of spinal cord, 8

Q
Quadriplegia Index of Function (QIF), 17
Quality of life, outcome measures of, 20–21
Quality of Life Index-SCI Version (SQL-SCI), 20
Quantitative sensory testing (QST), 16
Quebec User Evaluation of Satisfaction with Assistive Technology (QUEST), 21

R
Radiographic assessment, of acute spinal cord injury, 60t
Reaching, assistive technology for, 152–154, 153f, 155
Reactive oxygen species (ROS), 3–4
Rectal examination, 41

Rehabilitation, in spinal cord injury, 122. *See also* Assistive technology
  advanced strategies in, 163–178
    treadmill-based robotic devices, 164–168, 165*f*, 166*f*
    upper limb passive support systems, 173–174, 173*f*
    wearable sensors, 174–175, 175*f*, 176
  functional electrical stimulation (FES) therapy use in, 154–160
Reliability, of outcome measures, 11–12
Research, in spinal cord injury, 12–16
ReWalk™, 169–170, 169*f*
REX exoskeleton device, 171
Rick Hansen Spinal Cord Injury Registry, 86
Riluzole, neuroprotective effects of, 4, 80, 94*t*, 97, 104

S
Satisfaction with Life Scale (SWLS), 20
Schwann cells, in spinal cord injury, 90*f*–91*f*
Self-assembling peptides, 109*t*, 117
Sensorimotor rhythm (SRM)-based brain-computer interfaces, 181–182, 188–189
Sensors, wearable, 174–175, 175*f*, 176
Serum biomarkers, for functional recovery prediction, 25–38, 28*f*–30*f*
  structural biomarkers, 27–33, 28*t*–29*t*, 36*t*, 37
Shock, spinal, 41, 59
Short Form 36 (SF-36), 20
S100β, as spinal cord injury biomarker, 29*t*, 32, 37
Spasticity, diagnosis and assessment of, 21
Spectrin breakdown products, as spinal cord injury biomarkers, 32, 37
Spinal cord, complete transection of, 1–2
Spinal Cord Assessment Tool for Spastic reflexes (SCATS), 21
Spinal cord compression
  magnetic resonance imaging of, 40, 42–43, 54
  maximum (MSCC), 44, 45*t*, 46*f*
Spinal Cord Independence Measure (SCIM), 17
Spinal cord injury
  complications/consequences of, 57, 80
  incidence, 1, 80, 179
  incomplete, 122
  initial management of, 57–59, 59*t*–63*t*
  nonoperative management of, 57–70
  nontraumatic, outcome measures for, 22
  pathobiology of, 1–10, 132, 133*f*
    implication for surgical intervention, 71–72
  primary phase, 1–2, 2*t*, 8, 9, 57, 58*f*, 71, 72
  secondary phase, 1, 2–9, 2*t*, 3*f*, 57, 58*f*, 71, 72, 104
    acute, 2*t*, 3, 3*f*, 6, 72
    chronic, 2*t*, 3*f*
    effect of early surgical decompression on, 72–79
    implication for neuroprotective strategies, 89, 90*f*–92*f*
    intermediate chronic, 90*f*–91*f*

    primary/intermediate acute, 90*f*–91*f*
    subacute, 2*t*, 3*f*, 6, 72, 90*f*–91*f*
    without radiographic abnormality (SCIWORA), 62*t*
Spinal Cord Injury Functional Ambulatory Profile (SCI-FAP), 18
Spinal Cord Injury Pain Instrument (SCIPI), 19
Spinal Cord Outcomes Partnership Endeavor (SCOPE), 13, 21
Spinal Cord Research Evidence (SCIRE), 13, 21
Spinal cord trauma centers, 59
Standing
  epidural stimulation-assisted, 152
  functional electrical stimulation-assisted, 150
Steady-state evoked potential (SSEP)-based brain-computer interfaces, 181
Stem cells, of spinal cord, 8. *See also* Neural stem cell-based therapies
Step counters, 174
StepWatch Activity Monitor, 174
Stroke patients, brain-computer interface technology for, 157
Subaxial injuries, 61*t*
Surgical intervention, for spinal cord injury. *See* Decompression, surgical
Surgical Timing in Acute Spinal Cord Injury Study (STASCIS), 73, 80, 83, 85, 85*t*, 95

T
Tau protein, as spinal cord injury biomarker, 29*t*, 32–33
Tetraplegia, 179
Thoracic spine injury, early surgical decompression of, 73–74
Thoracolumbar spine injury, early surgical decompression of, 73–74
Thyrotropin-releasing hormone, neuroprotective effects of, 98
Timed Up and Go (TUG) test, 17
Tirilazad mesylate, neuroprotective effects of, 94*t*
Treadmill-based robotic devices, 164–168, 165*f*, 166*f*
  Aretech ZeroG®, 164–166, 166*f*
  Gait Trainer GT1, 167
  Lokomat®, 164, 165*f*
  LOwer extremity Powered ExoSkeleton (LOPES), 167–168
  PAM/POGO, 168
Tumor necrosis factor (TNF), as spinal cord injury biomarker, 30*t*, 34, 37

U
UCH-L1(ubiquitin carboxy-terminal hydrolase-L1), as spinal cord injury biomarker, 29*t*, 33, 37
Upper extremity
  exoskeleton devices for, 167–168, 172–174, 173*f*
  functional assessment of, 18–19, 22
  neuroprothesis control of, 184–185, 186*f*
  passive support system for, 173–174, 173*f*
  robotic trainers for, 172–174

V

Validity, of outcome measures, 11–12
Van Lieshout Test-Short Version (VLT-SV), 18–19
Vascular dysfunction, spinal cord injury-related, 57
Vasopressors, 59
Venous thromboembolism, prophylaxis for, 63*t*
Vertebral artery injury, 62*t*–63*t*
   magnetic resonance angiography of, 40, 44, 54
Viral vectors, of retrograde gene delivery, 103–104

W

Walking
   epidural stimulation-assisted, 152
   functional assessment of, 17–18, 22
   functional electrical stimulation-assisted,
      150–152, 151*f*, 154–155
   motorized lower extremity exoskeletons for, 184

   treadmill-based training devices for, 164–168,
      165*f*, 166*f*
   wearable robotic devices for, 168–172, 169*f*,
      171*f*
Walking Index of Spinal Cord Injury version 2
   (WISCI II), 17–18
Wartenberg Pendulum Test, 21
Wheelchair control, brain-computer interfaces for,
   183–184
Wings for Life (WfL) Spinal Cord Research Foun-
   dation, 48
World Health Organization (WHO), International
   Classification of Functioning, Disability and
   Health, 12

X

X-rays, role in trauma protocols, 40